IIW Collection

Series editor

Cécile Mayer, Villepinte, France

About the Series

The IIW Collection of Books is authored by experts from the 59 countries participating in the work of the 23 Technical Working Units of the International Institute of Welding, recognized as the largest worldwide network for welding and allied joining technologies.

The IIW's Mission is to operate as the global body for the science and application of joining technology, providing a forum for networking and knowledge exchange among scientists, researchers and industry.

Published books, Best Practices, Recommendations or Guidelines are the outcome of collaborative work and technical discussions-they are truly validated by the IIW groups of experts in joining, cutting and surface treatment of metallic and non-metallic materials by such processes as welding, brazing, soldering, thermal cutting, thermal spraying, adhesive bonding and microjoining. IIW work also embraces allied fields including quality assurance, non-destructive testing, standardization, inspection, health and safety, education, training, qualification, design and fabrication.

More information about this series at http://www.springer.com/series/13906

Bertil Jonsson · G. Dobmann
A.F. Hobbacher · M. Kassner
G. Marquis

IIW Guidelines on Weld Quality in Relationship to Fatigue Strength

INTERNATIONAL INSTITUTE OF WELDING
A world of joining experience

Springer

Bertil Jonsson
Hauler Loader Division
VOLVO Construction Equipment
Braås
Sweden

G. Dobmann
Fraunhofer—IZFP
Saarbrücken
Germany

A.F. Hobbacher
University of Applied Sciences
Wilhelmshaven
Germany

M. Kassner
ALSTOM Transport Deutschland GmbH
Salzgitter
Germany

G. Marquis
Department of Applied Mechanics
Aalto University
Espoo
Finland

ISSN 2365-435X ISSN 2365-4368 (electronic)
IIW Collection
ISBN 978-3-319-19197-3 ISBN 978-3-319-19198-0 (eBook)
DOI 10.1007/978-3-319-19198-0

Library of Congress Control Number: 2016936442

Printed on acid-free paper

This Springer imprint is published by Springer Nature
The registered company is Springer International Publishing AG Switzerland

Contents

Nomenclature

Cold lap	A region of non-fused overlap between the weld metal and base plate which results in an imperfection parallel to the base plate
Effective notch stress	Elastic notch stress calculated for a notch with a certain assumed notch radius
FAT	All fatigue resistance data including the FAT classes are given as characteristic values, which are assumed to represent a survival probability of at least 95 %, calculated from mean value on the basis of a two-sided 75 % tolerance limits of the mean. Other existing definitions, e.g., a survival probability of 95 % on the basis of 95 % one-sided limit of the mean or means minus two standard deviations corresponding to a survival probability of 97.7 %, are practically equal for engineering applications. Levels are arranged in steps
Geometric stress	See structural stress
Improved welds	Welds for which the weld toe is treated after welding by a grinding, re-melting, or peening operation. IIW Guidelines for select post-weld treatment methods have been published
Inclusion	Non-metallic material entrapped in molten metal during solidification
High quality weld	Welds with a lower level of imperfections such that it has fatigue strength greater than that defined in the IIW Guidelines and Recommendations with respect to nominal stress, hot spot stress, or effective notch stress. The improvement in fatigue strength is normally two FAT classes
Hot spot stress	See structural stress
k_m	Stress magnification factor for misalignment
Micro lack of fusion	Same as cold lap, used in some standards

Normal quality weld	Welds for which the level of imperfections is such that it satisfies the fatigue strength requirement defined in the IIW Guidelines and Recommendations with respect to nominal stress, hot spot stress, or effective notch stress
Notch stress	See effective notch stress
Overlap	A protrusion of weld metal beyond the weld toe or weld root. An overlap may be fused or non-fused. A toe overlap without fusion between the weld metal and base plate is the same as a cold lap
Porosity	Porosity is used to describe cavities or pores caused by gas entrapment in molten metal during solidification
N_f	Cycles to failure
Slag inclusion	See inclusion
Structural stress	A stress in a component, resolved to take into account the effects of a structural discontinuity on the surface of a hot spot, consisting of membrane and shell-bending stress components
Undercut	An unfilled groove along the fusion line between weld metal and base plate
ΔS or $\Delta\sigma$	Nominal stress range
ΔS_c or $\Delta\sigma_c$	Characteristic nominal stress range in MPa (see FAT above), but is a continuous variable when FAT are given in steps

Throat Thicknesses

Term	IIW terminology	Figure
Throat thickness	Thickness of a fillet weld	
Design throat thickness	Throat thickness specified by the designer	*Note* See Fig. 13 in ISO 17659
Nominal throat thickness	Design value of the height of the largest isosceles triangle that can be inscribed in the section of a fillet weld	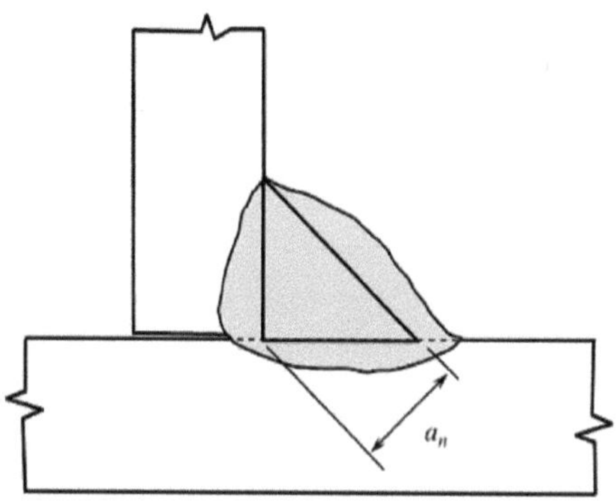 convex weld profile

(continued)

(continued)

Term	IIW terminology	Figure
		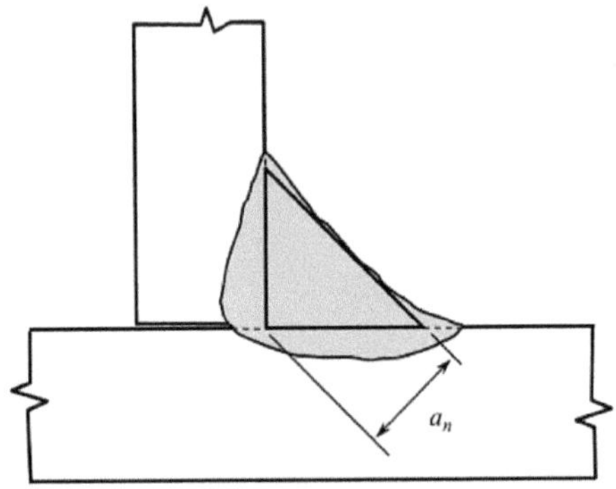 concave weld profile
Actual throat thickness	Throat thickness of the finalized weld measured according to the design throat thickness	The actual throat thicknesses will depend on whether the nominal throat thickness or effective throat thickness is used in design
Effective throat thickness	Design value of the height of the largest triangle that can be inscribed in the section of a fillet weld	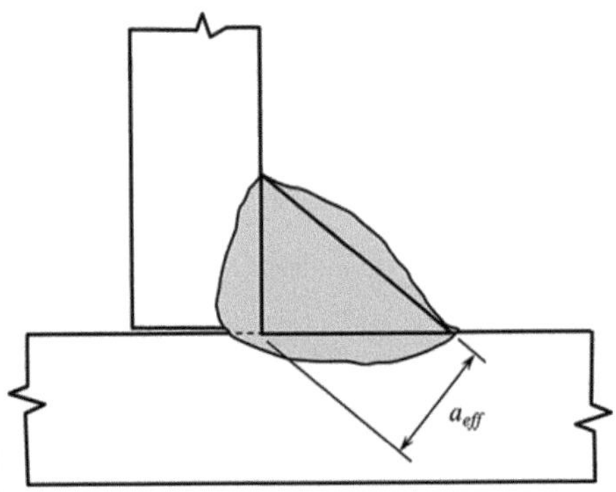

(continued)

(continued)

Term	IIW terminology	Figure
Maximum throat thickness	Nominal throat thickness to which a maximum amount of fusion penetration is added	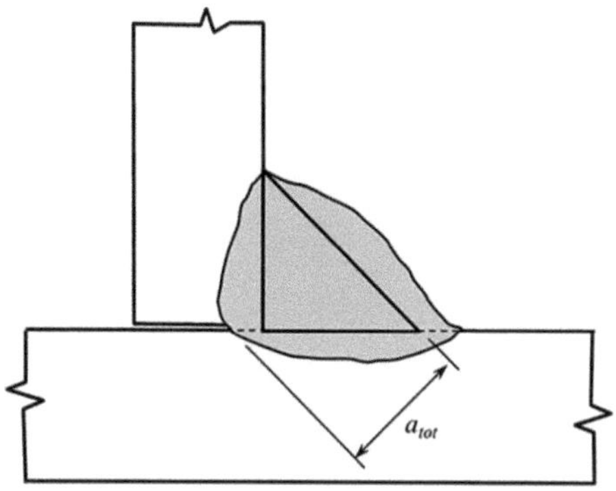
Utilized throat thickness	Effective throat thickness to which a certain amount of penetration is added	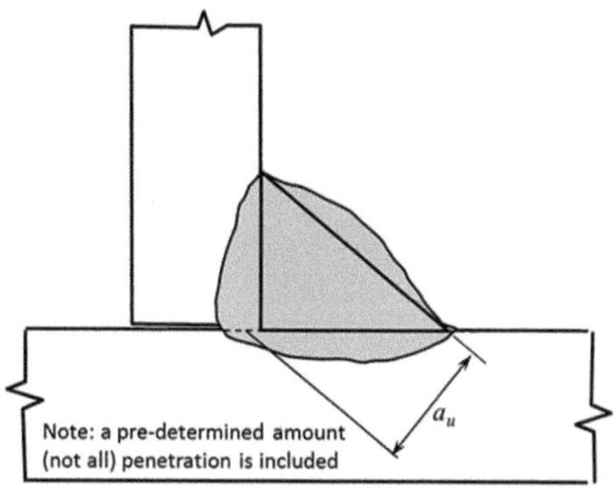

Note that other definitions may exist, the above-given are according to IIW, Commission VI

Chapter 1
Introduction

1.1 Existing IIW Recommendations and Guidelines

Complex welded structures are frequently exposed to demanding fatigue loading during service. In recent years, the Commission XIII of the International Institute of Welding (IIW) has developed several documents related to the analysis and design of welded structures to resist fatigue failure. These documents are intended to be fully consistent with one another and are intended to give well-defined methods which can serve as a basis for the fatigue design and assessment of welded components and structures subjected to fluctuating loads. They provide detailed guidelines for assessing both fatigue actions and the relevant fatigue resistance. The recommended methods include fatigue assessment based on nominal stress, structural stress, effective notch stress, linear elastic fracture mechanics, or laboratory testing.

- IIW Recommendations for Fatigue Design of Welded Joints and Components [1].
- Fatigue Analysis of Welded Components—Designer's guide to structural hot spot stress approach [2].
- IIW Guideline for the Fatigue Assessment by Notch Stress Analysis of Welded Structures [3].
- IIW Recommendations on Post-Weld Fatigue Life Improvement of Steel and Aluminum Structures [4].

This current guideline is intended to be used in connection with the previous referenced documents.

IIW guidelines and recommendations have been developed based on extensive laboratory testing combined with analytical and numerical modeling. Even a casual examination of background data which was used to develop these documents reveals that, for a given applied nominal stress range, the difference in fatigue life between the "weakest" and the "strongest" component is frequently one decade or more even for nominally identical test pieces. It is well established that these differences are the result of local geometric features of the weld bead, microscopic

B. Jonsson et al., *IIW Guidelines on Weld Quality in Relationship to Fatigue Strength*, IIW Collection, DOI 10.1007/978-3-319-19198-0_1

features of the weld toe, weld penetration, test piece misalignment, and residual stresses. No single geometric feature or imperfection type fully explains the resulting fatigue strength, but, rather, the combination and interaction of features is critical.

The intention of the current guideline is to provide quantitative and qualitative measures of geometric features and imperfections of a weld to ensure that it meets the fatigue strength demands found in the IIW Recommendations. Welds found to meet these quality requirements can be assessed in accordance with existing IIW Recommendations based on nominal stress [1], structural stress [2], or notch stress [3]. A second goal is to define a more restrictive acceptance criteria based on weld geometry features and imperfections which have increased fatigue strength. Fatigue strength for these welds is defined as S–N curves expressed in terms of nominal applied stress or hot spot stress. Where appropriate, reference is made to existing quality systems for welds, i.e., ISO 5817 [5] or Volvo's STD 181-0001 and 181-0004, where acceptance limits are given for different quality levels.

In addition to the acceptance criteria and fatigue assessment curves, guidance on their inspection and quality control are also given. Successful implementation of these methods depends on adequate training of operators as well as inspectors. It is anticipated that publication of the present IIW Recommendations will encourage the production of appropriate training aids and guidance for educating, training, and certifying operators and inspectors.

1.2 Scope

The Guidelines in the current document have been developed for fusion (arc and/or beam welding) welded steel plate-type structures. Plate thickness is assumed to be greater than 3 mm. Fatigue assessment is assumed to be based on either the nominal stress approach or structural stress approach as defined by the IIW Recommendations [1, 2]. More refined fatigue assessment based on notch stress concepts or fracture mechanics already included the ability to completely or partially account for weld geometric features and imperfections and are not specifically covered by this guideline.

It is assumed that the user has a working knowledge of the basics of fatigue and fracture mechanics. In some cases, working knowledge of finite element analysis is also needed. The recommendations and guidelines are considered to reflect the fatigue strength of the welded joint itself with a defined survival probability but without environmental effects. They are thus applicable to many industrial sectors. It is assumed that the user will apply good principals of limit state structural design. Appropriate partial safety factors for load and resistance must be applied depending on the industry.

The Guidelines apply to any arc-welded steel structure that is subjected to fatigue loading. Due to lack of experimental data for aluminum welds and ultra-high-strength steels, the fatigue strength (or S–N) curves apply only to structural steel up to a maximum specified yield strength of 960 MPa. However, it is reasonable to expect that acceptance criteria in the guideline would also be applicable to higher strength steels, stainless steels and that certain concepts would be applicable to 5000 and 6000 series aluminum alloys which are commonly used in welded structures. In the absence of relevant published data, it is recommended that such benefit should be quantified by special testing.

References

1. Hobbacher, A. (Editor): Recommendations for fatigue design of welded joints and components. IIW document XIII-2151-07/XV-1254-07. Welding Research Council New York, WRC-Bulletin 520, 2009
2. Fatigue analysis of welded components / designers guide to hot spot stress approach, IIW doc XIII-1819-00 / XV-1090-01 update 2003, Woodhead Publishing UK 2006 by Niemi E., Fricke W. & Maddox S.
3. Guideline for the fatigue assessment by notch stress analysis for welded structures, IIW document XIII-2240-08/XV-1289-08, 2008 By Fricke W.
4. Haagensen P.J. and Maddox S.J.: IIW Recommendations for weld toe improvement by grinding,TIG dressing and hammer peening for steel and aluminium structures.IIW doc. XIII-1815-00 (rev. 24 Feb. 2006)
5. ISO 5817:2006; Welding – Fusion-welded joints in steel, nickel, titanium and their alloys (beam welding excluded) – Quality levels for imperfections (ISO 5817:2003 +Cor. 1:2006), April 2006

Chapter 2
Design for Purpose

2.1 Limit State Design

Typical fabricated structures may have hundreds or even thousands of meters of weld. Thus, many potential fatigue cracking locations are present that must be considered during design development and production. The challenge is to optimize a design so that the welds have sufficient fatigue strength and fabrication quality to withstand the loads during the economic life of the structure or piece of equipment. Quality systems for welds are described in the so-called weld class systems, such as ISO 5817 or Volvo's old STD 181-0001. In these systems, acceptance limits are given for different weld geometry features or imperfections. Based on these limits, a weld is associated with a quality level, e.g., B, C, or D. Intuitively, a high-quality level, B, is assumed to perform better during the service than a weld with a C or D quality level. The problem with the existing weld quality systems is that they were initially developed as a measure of workmanship with respect to fabrication, i.e., as a measure of the skill of the individual or machine performing the operation. As such, they have been incorporated into a number of training and education programs for welders and weld inspectors. Numerous studies have shown that the link between the existing weld quality classes and fatigue performance is not consistent. Some acceptance criteria for some weld features or imperfections are found to have little or no influence on fatigue strength. For features which do influence fatigue strength, the acceptance criteria between quality classes do not result in uniform changes in the fatigue strength. Realizing that fatigue is highly affected by the local geometric features and imperfections of the weld, systems such as ISO 5817 could have been a good tool for quality measures regarding fatigue.

Designers of welded structures, on the other hand, think of weld quality in terms of performance. In this realm, quality would mean that a weld is able to perform its required function during the economic life of the component or structure. The required function may be major such as resistance to fatigue failure, sufficient strength with respect to extreme loads, impermeability, or corrosion resistance; or the

B. Jonsson et al., *IIW Guidelines on Weld Quality in Relationship to Fatigue Strength*, IIW Collection, DOI 10.1007/978-3-319-19198-0_2

required function could be a minor functional property such as hardness, resistance to abrasion, visual appearance, or surface finish. This way of thinking is consistent with modern design guidelines for structures which are based on limit state design considerations. One important feature of limit state design is the existence of clearly identified conditions or limits that constitute failure or feasibility for a structure. For a designer, any discussion of quality must relate the definition of weld quality with the limit state(s) that quantify failure. Fatigue strength is one of the most demanding limit state design criteria for welded structures.

2.2 Fatigue Versus Static Loading

The characteristic of the predominant load on the component is a major guiding consideration when formulating quality guidelines for load-carrying structures. For predominantly statically loaded welds, design calculations are based on the average stress in the weld net area. For this reason, ductility of the heat-affected zone (HAZ) and weld metal and sufficient weld throat thickness are the most important features. Imperfections such as porosity, undercuts, or cold laps have very little influence on the static capacity as long as the weld is ductile and the imperfections are small enough so as not to unexpectedly reduce the weld cross-sectional area. Thus, the ISO 5817 guideline includes many acceptance criteria which are not relevant for static loaded joints. Throat thickness is by far the most significant geometric feature of a weld subjected to predominantly static loading. Weld type (butt, fillet, V, K) does not significantly influence the strength for equal throat thickness.

Ductility and throat thickness are ensured by preproduction tests to validate the welding procedure specification (WPS). The same specification should ensure that crack-like imperfections are not formed during welding. For welded structures in high-strength steel, matching or overmatching of the weld metal strength may be difficult to achieve. In this case, insufficient static strength of the filler material can be compensated by adding filler material. Loss of ductility, however, cannot always be compensated for by adding material so this is considered to be the most important basic requirement of welding. Joint ductility is assumed in all types of structural durability assessment. The WPS provides a guideline which ensures the deformation capacity and strength of the joint. Thus, when defining the welding parameters, it is important to prioritize those parameters that produce required quality. Following this, aspects which improve productivity can be considered. Some structures will naturally have only very low load-carrying requirements, and in these cases, optimization of production costs can bring significant savings for fabrication. One example of this type of weld may be, for example, long fixing welds in statically loaded structures.

For predominantly fatigue loaded structures, the demands of ductility and sufficient throat thickness must obviously be maintained. But, because fatigue strength is significantly influenced by the local characteristics of the joint, extra requirements with respect to weld geometry and imperfections are imposed. In addition to throat thickness and ductility, Jonsson et al., for example, identified seven additional weld

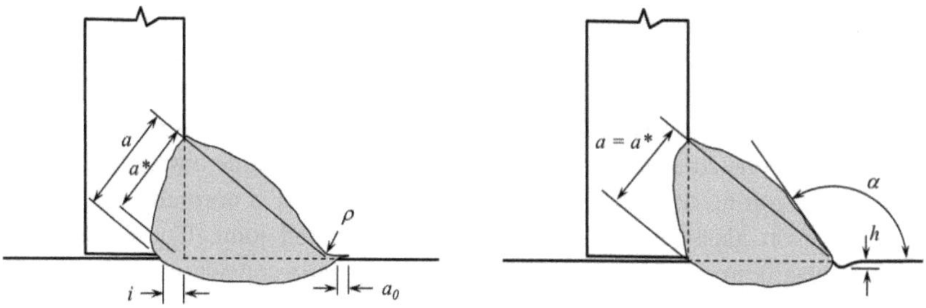

Fig. 2.1 Fillet weld geometry features which significantly influence fatigue strength. a Throat thickness, a^* fillet size, h depth of undercut, i weld penetration, ρ weld toe radius, a_0 cold lap length, and α weld angle

features which strongly influence fatigue strength: penetration, cold lap size, inner lack of fusion, weld toe transition radius, undercut size, joint misalignment, and porosity (see Fig. 2.1). It can be noted that in some technical literature, the cold lap imperfection shown in Fig. 2.1 is sometimes referred to as a micro-lack of fusion or a non-fused overlap. In technical literature, there is some inconsistency as to the definition of throat thickness, a, for partially penetrated welds. In this document, the definition is consistent with the Eurocodes, i.e., weld throat thickness includes also the penetration. The fillet size, a^*, is defined as being measured from the intersection of the plates as shown in Fig. 2.1. Thus, for fillet welds with no penetration, $a = a^*$; and for fillet welds with penetration, $a \approx a^* + i/\sqrt{2}$. Porosity is categorized based on pore location, diameter, and whether the pores occur singly or as a cluster. Weld angle can have an influence on fatigue strength. However, for fillet welds with high fatigue strength, weld angle is far less important than weld toe radius. For welds which have fatigue strength meeting IIW Recommendations, $\alpha \geq 90°$ is sufficient.

Root side fatigue can be the result of poor design or improper WPS. If a full penetration weld is not designated, lack of penetration may serve as a large initial defect. The greater the defect, the shorter the expected life so the root side fatigue strength can vary from near zero to a value far exceeding the fatigue strength of the weld toe or plate edge. Designing against fatigue is thus strongly dependent on the needed weld penetration. This value is determined by analysis using the effective notch method, fracture mechanics, or other suitable method. It is suggested that root side penetration be specified on the production drawing and that the quality requirement is simply that penetration is equal to or greater than this value.

2.3 Weld Quality and Design

Weld quality with respect to fatigue is controlled largely based on the local geometry of the weld toe. In any single welded joint, there may be numerous fatigue critical locations depending on the weld type and direction of loading.

In multipass welding, the notches occurring between beads can also be critical. If weld quality is limited to include only the weld toe geometry, it means that quality is controlled by the fabrication processes. Factors other than weld geometry that relate to the fabrication phase and that possibly affect the strength of the joint must be taken into consideration by the designer during the fatigue assessment process. For example, during design, the structural hot spot stress is normally calculated on the basis of an idealized and perfectly aligned welded joint. Consequently, any possible misalignment has to be taken explicitly into consideration in the FEA model or by applying an appropriate stress magnification factors k_m. This applies particularly to butt welds, cruciform joints, and one-sided transverse fillet-welded attachments on one side of unsupported plates.

Table 2.1 summarizes the relationships between the most common fatigue assessment methods and weld imperfections or misalignment. The nominal stress method partially addresses both imperfections and misalignment in the fatigue resistance (S–N) curves. The hot spot stress and notch stress S–N curves were developed for welds representing typical workshop quality. The notch stress method could be applied to some weld imperfection issues; for example, the influence of undercuts or pores could be modeled using a fictitious radius and the influence of weld angle can also be considered.

Angular distortion and misalignment errors shown in Fig. 2.2 do not fully belong to the quality level even though they occur during the welding process. The S–N curves for hot spot stress or notch stress already include a small magnification factor (5 %) for secondary stresses due to misalignment. The maximum degree of misalignment must be specified by the designer and taken into account as additional

Table 2.1 Relations between fatigue assessment methods, imperfections, and misalignments

<table>
<tr><th>Fatigue assessment method</th><th>Imperfections</th><th>Misalignment</th></tr>
<tr><td>Nominal stress</td><td>Some imperfection acceptance limits are specified for some joint types</td><td>Acceptance limits are specified for different joint types—additional misalignment must be computed by magnifying factor for the fatigue action</td></tr>
<tr><td>Structural stress</td><td>Normal workmanship imperfections are included in the fatigue resistance (S–N) curve</td><td rowspan="3">Up to 5 % increase in stress is included in the fatigue resistance (S–N) curve—additional misalignment must be computed by magnifying factor for the fatigue action</td></tr>
<tr><td>Notch stress</td><td>Normal workmanship imperfections are included in the fatigue resistance (S–N) curve—some other imperfection types, e.g., large undercut could be modeled</td></tr>
<tr><td>Linear fracture mechanics</td><td>Normal workmanship imperfections are included in the Paris law data—some other imperfection types, e.g., large pores could be modeled</td></tr>
</table>

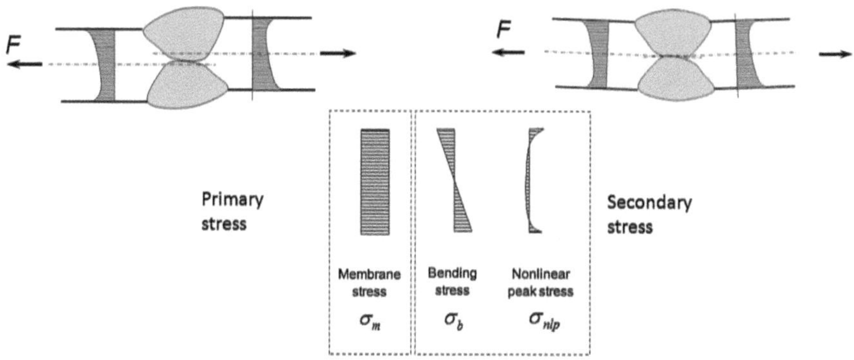

Fig. 2.2 Angular distortion and misalignment imperfections in butt welds

structural stress loading. This is a departure from current practice, but the procedure is analogous to considering the additional structural stress concentration produced by the step effect from butt-welded joints between plates of different thicknesses. The designer should be concerned about this kind of imperfection and should determine the permissible structural asymmetries for different types of loading. If maximum misalignment is not specified, then values found in the IIW Recommendations for nominal stress-based fatigue assessment should be used.

2.4 Practical Design for Purpose

Based on the type of loading, differentiation must be made between various joint categories. Design criteria and quality requirements will depend heavily on the primary function of the joint. Applied loads and structural geometry together establish the joint function. The simple welded T-joints shown in Fig. 2.3 can have numerous functions based on the applied forces, F1–F4.

If the joint is loaded by the force component F1, the weld is a shear-loaded longitudinal weld. Web-to-flange welds in plate girders are typical examples of this type of weld. In such cases, the acceptance criteria related to the weld toe are rarely significant, but failure from the weld root may occur.

For the longitudinal weld loaded by F2, weld start and stop positions become critical and the waviness of the fusion line may have strong influence on fatigue strength. If the joint is loaded by the force component F3, the weld is a non-load-carrying accessory weld and the weld toe geometry at the base plate to weld fusion line becomes crucial, i.e., cold lap size, weld toe transition radius, and undercut size. Welds loaded by F3 can also be considered as moderately demanding with respect to fabrication. A non-loaded accessory weld will never be critical in static loading cases but will often lead to fatigue failure.

For load-carrying fillet welds subjected to F4, the weld toe geometry at the attachment-to-weld fusion line is critical. Cold lap size, inner lack of fusion, weld

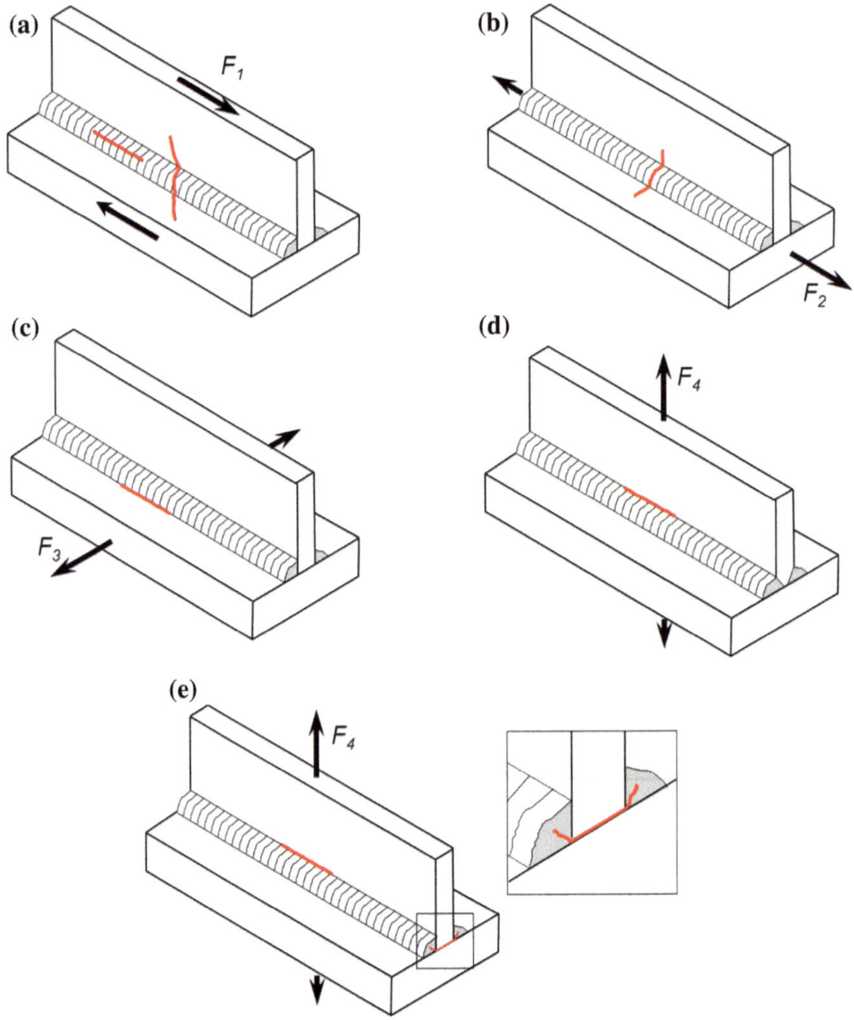

Fig. 2.3 Joint classification is determined based on joint loading/function: **a** longitudinal shear-loaded fillet weld, **b** longitudinal normal-loaded fillet weld, **c** transverse normal non-load-carrying fillet weld, **d** transverse normal load-carrying fillet weld, toe cracking, and **e** transverse load-carrying fillet weld, root cracking. *Red lines* indicate fatigue critical points

toe transition radius, undercut size, joint misalignment porosity, and weld penetration all potentially have strong influence on the fatigue strength of the joint. For a weld loaded with force F4, a root side fatigue crack may also develop depending on the degree of penetration. Welds loaded by F4 are the most demanding both with respect to design and fabrication because both the weld toe side and root side must be considered.

Chapter 3
IIW Fatigue Assessment Procedures

Numerous fatigue assessment methods have been introduced to assess the durability of metal structures under dynamic loading. Finite element (FE) modeling is an integral part of most design and analysis work, and methods have evolved as the analysis possibilities have become more sophisticated and computers have increased in speed and memory capacity. Fatigue assessment places two conflicting demands on the analysts. The fatigue damage process itself is highly local, thus requiring a fine FE mesh. On the other hand, welded structures are frequently large and geometrically complex, they have numerous load input locations, and they have boundary conditions which may be difficult to define. These demands are best satisfied with a large FE model. Because of this conflict, fatigue assessment is frequently the slowest link in the design process of welded structures.

The fatigue resistance and fatigue life of welded joints can be evaluated based on fatigue testing, the nominal stress method, the hot spot method, the notch stress/strain method, or crack growth simulations based on linear elastic fracture mechanics. The different assessment methods are described in detail in the IIW recommendations on fatigue. A short overview of these methods is given in Sect. 5.1. The different assessment methods are described in detail in the IIW recommendations on fatigue (Ref. [1] in Chap. 1) and will not be repeated here.

3.1 Available Assessment Procedures

3.1.1 Fatigue Testing

The most precise method to derive information about a welded component or structure is to perform comparative experimental tests. Virtually, all of the fatigue assessment procedures available have been developed and verified based on extensive experimental testing. However, there may be interest and justification for

B. Jonsson et al., *IIW Guidelines on Weld Quality in Relationship to Fatigue Strength*, IIW Collection, DOI 10.1007/978-3-319-19198-0_3

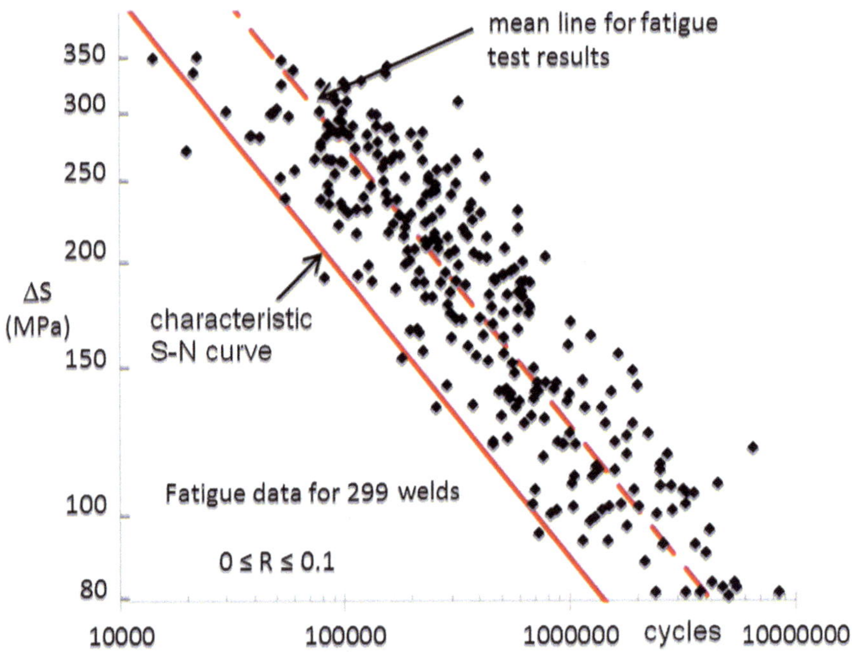

Fig. 3.1 Typical scatter observed during fatigue testing of welded components

experimental evaluation, e.g., for verifying new designs, for optimizing a fabrication procedure, or for assessing potential unexpected failure modes.

Experimental test results must be evaluated by sound statistical methods. There is often a special problem when evaluating data collections from different laboratories. For example, nominally identical test components may differ systematically if they have been fabricated at different locations. There may also be variations in test fixture or test procedures which must be considered. Statistical assessment of welded components is normally based on the assumption of a lognormal distribution of the data with respect to stress range or fatigue life. When comparing test data to specific design lines, one must be aware that the design lines represent a very low probability of failure (see FAT of nomenclature above) and should be sufficiently conservative with respect to the test data (see Fig. 3.1, [ISO TR on testing, Ref. 2]). Also, in some cases, it may happen that the test results do not seem to follow the Gaussian lognormal distribution, then other distributions may be more relevant, one example often used is the Weibull distribution.

3.1.2 Nominal Stress Method

Most design guidance documents related to fatigue, such as IIW or Eurocode 3, are based on the nominal stress method. Stress computations based on this method are also relatively straightforward. These reasons make it the most widely used fatigue assessment method for welded structures. The nominal stress method provides satisfactory results for relatively little effort as long as the following conditions are met:

1. The nominal stress can be clearly defined and is not significantly influenced by macro-geometric effects which raise stress in the vicinity of the welded joint, e.g., large openings, beam curvature, and concentrated loads.
2. The structural discontinuity to be evaluated is geometrically comparable with one of the geometries defined in the fatigue design guidance document or standard.
3. The misalignments and/or welding defects in the joint are consistent with those defined in the fatigue design guidance document or standard.

Nominal stress is the stress calculated in the sectional area under consideration, disregarding the local stress-raising effects of the welded joint, but including the stress-raising effects of the macro-geometric shape of the component in the vicinity of the joint, such as large cutouts. Overall, elastic behavior is assumed.

The nominal stress S–N curves are derived based on extensive experimental testing. The IIW defines 12 curves for welded joints and one curve for base metal failure. The welded joint curves are valid for $N > 10^4$ cycles, and all have an inverse slope $m = 3$. Curves are defined by means of a FAT class which represents the stress range at $N = 2 \times 10^6$. At $N > 1 \times 10^7$, the slope changes to $m = 5$ for assessing variable amplitude loading and $m = 22$ for high-cycle constant amplitude loading. In the IIW fatigue recommendations, the so-called FAT classes represent characteristic fatigue strength values that correspond to a certain survival probability. The stress value is defined only in terms of stress range, and the welding residual stresses are assumed to be high. Given that FAT values are valid for thicknesses $t \leq 25$ mm, for higher t, a penalty factor is given, the so-called thickness effect. Special consideration must be given for $N < 104$ or for structures which are stress relieved or known to have low residual stresses (see Fig. 3.2).

The influence of mean stress which is very dramatic for base material fatigue is much less pronounced in the case of welded details. For thick plates or some large complex welded structures, the fabrication process or assembly constraint may produce large-scale or structural residual stresses which induce high local residual stresses in the region where fatigue cracks initiate and propagate and in these cases, no mean stress effect is recommended. For stress-relieved structures, the applied fatigue loads can be increased by a factor of:

$$1.6 \quad \text{for } R \leq -1 \text{ or if the applied loading is fully compressive}$$
$$1.2 - 0.4 * R \quad \text{for } -1 \leq R \leq 0.5$$

For small or thin-walled components without assembly constraint, the applied fatigue loads can be increased by a factor of:

$$1.3 \quad \text{for } R \leq -1 \text{ or if the applied loading is fully compressive}$$
$$0.9 - 0.4 * R \quad \text{for } -1 \leq R \leq -0.25$$

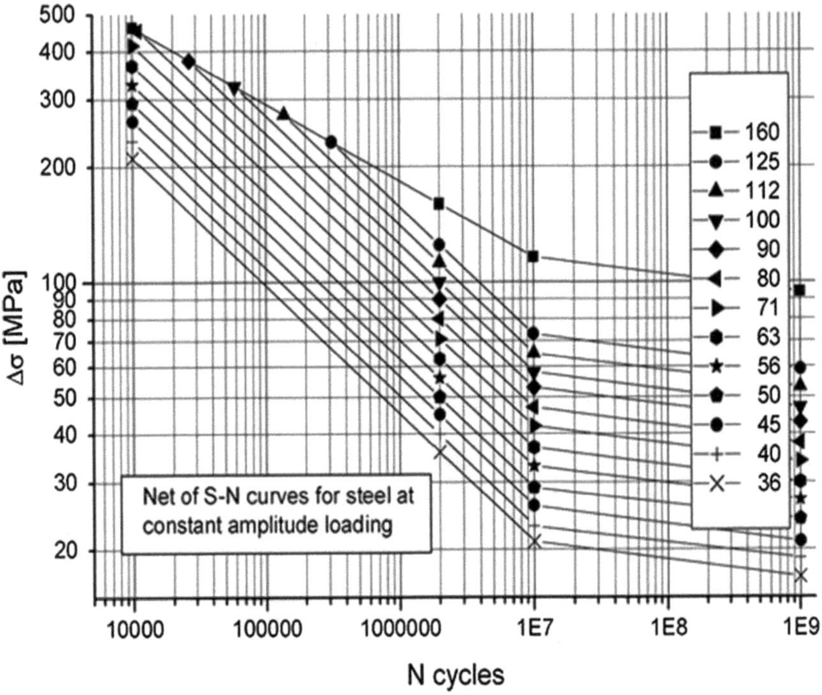

Fig. 3.2 S–N curves for constant amplitude fatigue loading of steel-welded joints

These factors are given by the IIW recommendations and have been validated for materials with yield strengths up to 960 MPa.

3.1.3 *Structural Hot Spot Stress Method*

The hot spot method is included in the new European standard, *EN 1993-1-9,* and in the most recent IIW recommendation, see Ref. [3]. In the hot spot stress method, two S–N curves are used for all structural discontinuities because the calculated hot spot stress already incorporates many of the stress-raising effects of the welded joint. This method is used mainly when the angle between the weld of the joint to be examined and the direction in which the stress fluctuates is more or less perpendicular, and it can be assumed that the crack will form on the weld toe. The method is not applicable for cases in which the crack grows from the root or from defects inside the weld. When compared with the nominal stress method, the hot spot method is more suitable in the following cases:

1. The nominal stress in the structure cannot be clearly determined due to its complex geometry,
2. The structural detail is not easily comparable with the any of the typical fatigue details presented in design guidance documents for the nominal stress method,
3. Finite element-based stress analyses of the structure have been performed, and/or strain gauge measurement results suitable for hot spot stress assessment are available for the structure or a prototype, or
4. The offset misalignment and/or angular misalignment of the joint exceed the limit values permitted by the nominal stress method.

In contrast to the nominal stress method where stresses are computed using simple strength of materials equations, the hot spot stress method requires a more complete understanding of stress components at a welded joint. With reference to Fig. 3.3, the stress through the wall of a plate is nonlinear and stress components can be separated. The three components are membrane stress, shell bending stress, and nonlinear peak stress. The structural stress comprises the sum of the membrane stress and shell bending stress. This sum is linearly distributed through the thickness of a plate. The hot spot stress is the value of this linear stress on the plate surface at the weld toe.

The hot spot stress can be determined experimentally based on surface extrapolation along the plate surface using strain gauges (see Fig. 3.4). However, the hot

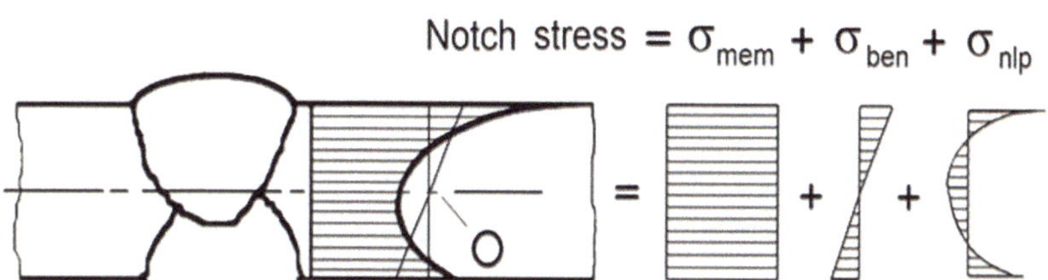

Fig. 3.3 Stress components at a weld

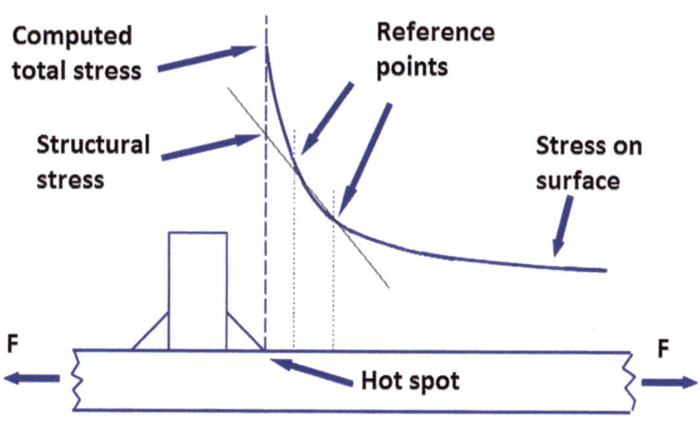

Fig. 3.4 Stress extrapolation to the weld toe to determine the hot spot stress

spot stress is normally determined based on finite element analysis (FEA) using either surface extrapolation to the weld toe or linearizing the through-the-thickness stresses at the weld toe. When using FEA, specific meshing recommendations including mesh size and element type should be followed. Fatigue assessment is based on the computed hot spot stress and either the FAT 90 or FAT 100 S–N line. The FAT 90 curve is used if the joint is non-load-carrying, while the FAT 100 curve is used for load-carrying or partial load-carrying joints.

The main drawback of the method is the limitation to weld toe failures and need to perform extrapolation which introduces some uncertainty. The designer has to verify that the welded joint will not fail from the root or inner defects. Disregarding these limitations, the method is well established in tubular structures, shipbuilding, and other areas of application and it is expected to gain more significance in the future.

3.1.4 Effective Notch Stress Method

FE analysis as a basis for fatigue design analysis of welded structures usually leads to problems related to the incompatibility of the stress results produced by FE analysis and those needed for the fatigue design procedures; i.e., nominal stresses are often difficult or impossible to define, structural stresses are determined by extrapolation techniques, and stress intensity factors are found, for example, by integration with special element types. In this respect, the effective notch stress approach has an advantage over the other methods in that the stress value used in analysis is unambiguous since it is the maximum computed stress at a well-defined location in the FE model (see Ref. [5]). The IIW has prepared guidelines for implementing the effective notch stress method in fatigue analysis of welded structures (see Ref. [4]).

The usual local-strain approach, see Ref. [4], cannot normally be applied directly to welded joints because the weld geometry always has some degree of irregularity, and strain-life material parameters at the weld toe are non-homogeneous and rarely available. The irregularity of the weld toe and the root configuration prevent from a normal determination of notch stress. More recent investigations have shown that the irregular notch at welded joints can be replaced by an effective one of a radius of 1 mm for plate thicknesses ≥5 mm (see Fig. 3.5). The results are consistent within the scatter usually observed at welded joints and can be used as a basis for a regulation by codes, which firstly was done here. With the rising performance of computing power, a growing application of the method is expected.

The effective notch stress may be determined by FE or boundary element analysis. Meshing procedures with respect to mesh size and element type should be strictly followed when applying this method. The assessment is then done by the use of a single S–N curve. For steel, the FAT 225 curve represents a high survival probability (see definition under nomenclature). Both the weld toe and weld root gap can be assessed using this curve. Note that the method computes something like a stress concentration factor, K_t, but the transition to the fatigue notch factor, K_f, is

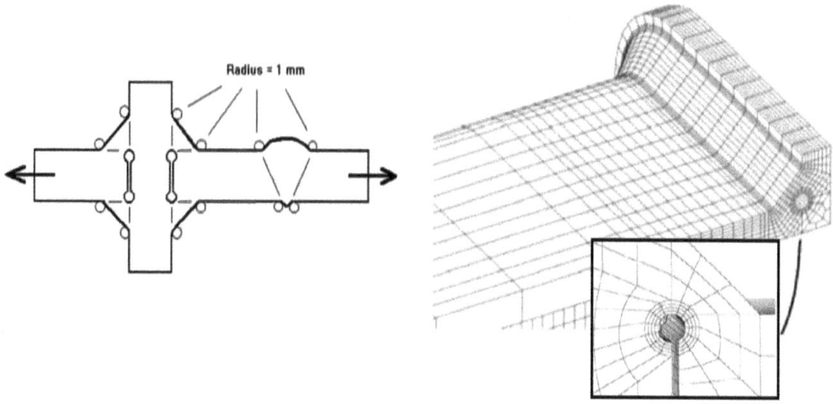

Fig. 3.5 The effective 1-mm-radius notch is used to model all potential fatigue crack initiation sites

implicitly included in the FAT value. Effects of weld toe angle, leg lengths, and undercut can be assessed as well, which is not possible at structural hot spot stress method. An effect of wall thickness is automatically covered by the notch stress, and the thickness effect does not need to be considered explicitly.

3.1.5 Fracture Mechanics Method

Since the welded components behave like severely notched or corroded ones with a short period of crack initiation, it is reasonable to consider the crack propagation as the governing process and to use fracture mechanics. The fracture mechanics concept is useful for the assessment of cracks or crack-like imperfections. The knowledge of the notch stress distribution in the vicinity of the crack is required, such as membrane, shell bending, and nonlinear peak stress. Furthermore, a formula for the determination of the stress intensity factor (SIF) is required. The fatigue life can be determined by integrating the *Paris–Erdogan* power law (Eq. 3.1).

$$\frac{da}{dN} = C_0 \cdot \Delta K^m \quad \text{for } \Delta K > K_{\text{th}} \text{ where } K = \sigma \cdot \sqrt{\pi \cdot a} \cdot Y(a) \cdot M_k(a) \tag{3.1}$$

Parametric formulae for the determination of the SIF have been developed for a multitude of structural details. They are based on well-established formulae for cracks in plates under membrane and shell bending stress. An additional function $M_k(a)$ considers the nonlinear stress peak and the special geometrical conditions of the different structural details and joint types. Here, the IIW recommendations give formulae and refer to selected literature. For further details, see Chap. 7.

The resistance against crack propagation under the load of cyclic stress intensity has been derived from earlier data collections and is given in Sect. 8.4 as the material parameters of the *Paris–Erdogan* power law of crack propagation.

For the assessment of crack-like imperfections, the initial dimensions of the imperfection have to be determined by nondestructive material testing methods.

The final crack size does not need to be determined precisely. If a crack grows to about one half of the wall thickness ($t/2$), the fatigue life is practically over. Most of the life is spent at small cracks, i.e., in the beginning of the growth. In critical cases, a check using the R6 method, see Ref. [1], for the assessment of the final rupture might be useful.

References

1. R6: Assessment of Integrity of Structures Containing Defects, Revision 4, 2001, including updates to amendment 8, 2010, British Energy Generation Ltd. Goucester
2. Recommendations on fatigue testing of welded joints, IIW Doc XIII-2114-06 by Lieurade, HP., Hutter M. & Maddox S
3. Fatigue analysis of welded components/ designers guide to hot spot stress approach, IIW doc XIII-1819-00/ XV-1090-01 update 2003, Woodhead Publishing UK 2006 by Niemi E., Fricke W. & Maddox S
4. Guideline for the fatigue assessment by notch stress analysis for welded structures, IIW document XIII-2240-08/XV-1289-08, 2008 By Fricke W
5. Fatigue assessment of welded joints by local approaches, 2nd edition, WP By Radaj D., Sonsino C.M., Fricke W

Chapter 4
Classification of Weld Imperfections and Features

The designation and the classification of weld imperfections and features depend on both the material being joined, e.g., steel or aluminum, and the joining process, e.g., fusion welding, pressure welding, etc.

4.1 Overview About Classifications of Weld Imperfections in ISO Standards

A general designation system for imperfections of welding and allied process is contained in ISO/TS 17845:2004 [1]. This ISO standard covers both metallic and nonmetallic materials. A classification of geometric imperfections in metallic materials is given for fusion welding in ISO 6520-1 [2] and for pressure welding in ISO 6520-2 [3]. Neither standard includes classifications for metallurgical imperfections.

The geometric weld imperfections for fusion welding in ISO 6520-1 are relevant for arc and beam welding processes covering metallic materials: steel, nickel, titanium, aluminum, and their alloys. This document contains the relevant classification of geometric imperfections for these welding processes, but no information about the relevant quality level or limits are provided.

Acceptance limits for the imperfections defined in EN ISO 6520-1 are given in order to define quality levels. For arc-welded joints (excluding beam welding) in steel, nickel, titanium and their alloys, quality levels are defined in ISO 5817 [4] and for aluminum and its alloys the quality levels are defined in ISO 10042 [5]. For electron- and laser-beam-welded joints in steel, quality levels are defined in ISO 13919-1 [6] and for aluminum and its alloys in ISO 13919-2 [7]. For laser-arc hybrid welding of steels, nickel, and nickel alloys, there are quality levels for imperfections ISO 12932:2013 [13].

B. Jonsson et al., *IIW Guidelines on Weld Quality in Relationship to Fatigue Strength*, IIW Collection, DOI 10.1007/978-3-319-19198-0_4

In these standards which define quality levels and limits, the following quality classes are used: quality class B refers to high-quality requirements, quality class C refers to middle-quality requirements, and quality class D refers to low-quality requirements.

The geometric weld imperfections for pressure-based welding processes, such as pressure butt welding, resistance spot welding, are given in ISO 6520-2. These are relevant for all metallic materials. In the relation of quality criteria for welded joints, the general tolerances for welded structures in ISO 13920 [8] should also be considered. The relevant imperfection standard for thermal cutting is ISO 9013 [9] and ISO 12584 (ISO 17658 [10]). For several new fusion welding processes, standards for relevant imperfections have not yet been adopted. These include friction stir welding.

4.2 Classification of Geometric Imperfections for Fusion Welds in Metallic Materials, ISO 6520-1

For fusion welding of metallic materials, ISO 6520-1 [2] contains a classification of all relevant geometric imperfections without direct information for quality requirements or limits. In this standard, there are 6 main groups of geometric imperfections:

- cracks (No. 100),
- cavities (No. 200),
- solid inclusions (No. 300),
- lack of fusion and penetration (No. 400),
- imperfect shape and dimension (No. 500),
- miscellaneous imperfection (No. 600).

These main groups consist of 45 main imperfections and 79 sub-imperfections.

Most of the main imperfections and some sub-imperfections of ISO 6520-1 are considered in the standards with direct information about the quality level and quality limit [4–7, 13]. Table 4.1 presents a sample of the overview of all imperfections of ISO 6520-1, for which there are quality limits in these standards. Furthermore, this table contains also information for these imperfections which are relevant both for butt welds and fillet welds and with respect to toe or root failure. The table also gives information about defect types which are not allowed in the weld quality standards or for which quantitative limits are specified and related to quality groups B, C, or D.

In ISO 6520-1, some of the imperfections are known to have a very strong influence on fatigue strength, but quantitative limits of these imperfections are not defined in the quality standards with imperfection limits [4–7, 13], e.g., incorrect weld toe radius (No. 5052 in ISO 6520-1) and angular misalignment (No. 508 in ISO 6520-1).

Table 4.1 Example of geometric imperfections in welded metallic materials according to ISO 6520-1 and their consideration in the standards with imperfection limits [4–7]

Geometric imperfection according to ISO 6520-1				Relevance for			Acceptance level of imperfection			
Main imperfection		Sub-imperfection		Butt weld	Fillet weld		Arc welding		Beam welding ISO 13919	
Ref. No.	Designation explanation	Ref. No.	Designation explanation		Toe	Root	Steel ISO 5817	Alum. ISO 10042	Steel part 1	Alum. part 2
202	Shrinkage cavity			X		X	D		D, C, B	D, C, B
	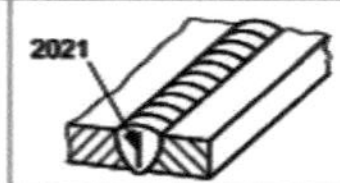	2021	Interdendritic shrinkage	X		X				
	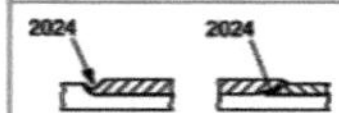	2024	Crater pipe	X		X	D		D, C, B	D, C, B
	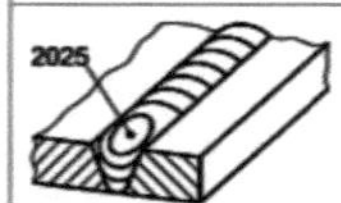	2025	End crater pipe	X		X	D	D, C		
300	Solid inclusion			X		X	D, C, B		No limit	D, C, B
302	Flux inclusion			X		X	D, C, B			
303	Oxide inclusion			X		X	D, C, B	D, C, B		
304	Metallic inclusion			X		X	D, C, B	D, C, B		
		3042	Copper	X		X	Not allowed			
400	Lack of fusion and penetration			X	X	X	D, C (outside)	D	D	D
401	Lack of fusion			X		X	D			
4011	Lack of sidewall fusion			X		X	D			

(continued)

Table 4.1 (continued)

Geometric imperfection according to ISO 6520-1				Relevance for			Acceptance level of imperfection			
Main imperfection		Sub-imperfection		Butt weld	Fillet weld		Arc welding		Beam welding ISO 13919	
Ref. No.	Designation explanation	Ref. No.	Designation explanation		Toe	Root	Steel ISO 5817	Alum. ISO 10042	Steel part 1	Alum. part 2
	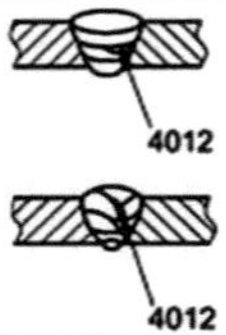	4012	Lack of inter-run fusion	X		X	D			
	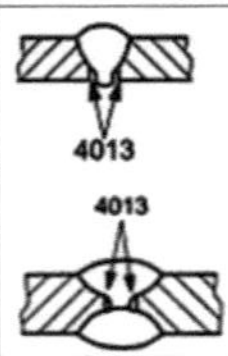	4013	Lack of root fusion	X		X	D			

Table 4.2 Number of considered imperfections in standards with quality limits

Weld process	Material	Standard	Surface imperfection	Inside imperfection	Imperfection of weld geometry	Superposition of different imperfections
Arc welding	Steel	ISO 5817	23	13	3	2
	Aluminum	ISO 10042	18	12	2	1
Beam welding	Steel	ISO 13919-1	18			
	Aluminum	ISO 13919-2	20			

On the other hand, the quality standards with imperfection limits [4–7, 13] also consider imperfections which are not included in ISO 6520-1. These additional imperfections are, for example, multiple imperfections (ISO 5817: No. 4.1 and 4.2; ISO 10042: 4.1) and deviation of penetration angle (ISO 13919-1 and ISO 13919-2: No. 17). Table 4.2 contains the number of the considered imperfections in the standards with imperfection limits [4–7, 13].

4.3 Quality Criteria of Welded Joints in ISO 5817

For arc welding of steel structures, the standard ISO 5817 contains detailed limits of imperfections related to the quality levels

- B: high-quality requirements,
- C: middle-quality requirements,
- D: low-quality requirements.

In this standard, there are no information about the relevance of imperfections for static and fatigue strength. Table 4.3 shows an excerpt of ISO 5817. Because arc welding of steel structures is a main application area of welded structures, this standard has dominant position for quality controls of welded joints. In ISO 5817, the imperfection limits are related to two thickness ranges of welded plates: thickness $0.5 \leq t \leq 3$ mm or thickness $t > 3$ mm.

The ISO 5817 contains the following:

- 23 outside imperfections (imperfections No. 1.1–1.23),
- 13 inside imperfections (imperfections No. 2.1–2.13),
- two weld geometry imperfections (imperfections No. 3.1 and 3.2),
- two types of multiple imperfections/superimposed imperfections (imperfections No. 4.1 and 4.2).

Table 4.3 Excerpt of ISO 5817

No.	Reference to ISO 6520-1:1998	Imperfection designation	Remarks	t mm	Limits for imperfections for quality levels D	C	B
1 Surface imperfections							
1.1	100	Crack	—	≥ 0,5	Not permitted	Not permitted	Not permitted
1.2	104	Crater crack	—	≥ 0,5	Not permitted	Not permitted	Not permitted
1.3	2017	Surface pore	Maximum dimension of a single pore for — butt welds — fillet welds	0,5 to 3	$d \leq 0,3\ s$ $d \leq 0,3\ a$	Not permitted	Not permitted
			Maximum dimension of a single pore for — butt welds — fillet welds	> 3	$d \leq 0,3\ s$, but max. 3 mm $d \leq 0,3\ a$, but max. 3 mm	$d \leq 0,2\ s$, but max. 2 mm $d \leq 0,2\ a$, but max. 2 mm	Not permitted
1.4	2025	End crater pipe	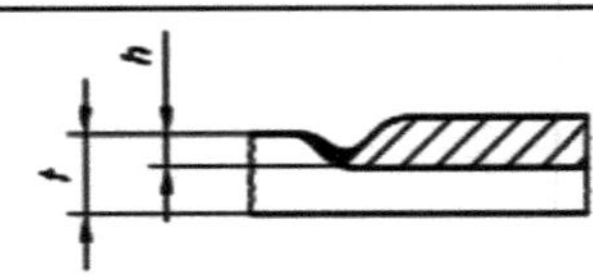	0,5 to 3	$h \leq 0,2\ t$	Not permitted	Not permitted
				> 3	$h \leq 0,2\ t$, but max. 2 mm	$h \leq 0,1\ t$, but max. 1 mm	Not permitted
1.5	401	Lack of fusion (incomplete fusion)	—	≥ 0,5	Not permitted	Not permitted	Not permitted
		Micro lack of fusion	Only detectable by micro examination		Permitted	Permitted	Not permitted
1.6	4021	Incomplete root penetration	Only for single side butt welds 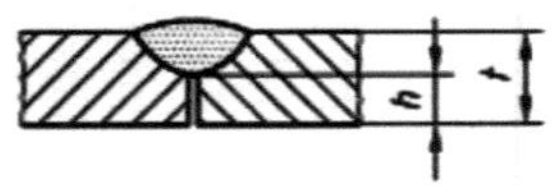	≥ 0,5	Short imperfections: $h \leq 0,2\ t$, but max. 2 mm	Not permitted	Not permitted

Table 4.4 Imperfections with limit information for quality level D, C, and B

Quality group	No. according to ISO 5817	Imperfection designation
Surface imperfections	1.7	Continuous and non-continuous undercut
	1.8	Root notch
	1.9	Excessive weld overfill
	1.10	Excessive convexity
	1.11	Excessive root overfill
	1.12	Incorrect weld toe
	1.14	Sagging, incomplete filled groove
	1.16	Excessive asymmetry
	1.17	Root concavity
	1.21	Excessive throat thickness
Internal imperfections	2.2	Micro-crack
	2.3	Pore porosity
	2.4	Pore net, clustered porosity
	2.5	Pore line
	2.6	Wormhole
	2.9	Solid inclusion, slag inclusion
	2.10	Metallic inclusion
Imperfections in joint geometry	3.1	Axial misalignment
	3.2	Incorrect root gap for fillet welds
Multiple imperfections	4.1	Multiple imperfections in any cross section
	4.2	Projected or cross-sectional area in longitudinal direction of weld

Some imperfections are only valid for butt welds and others for fillet welds. Furthermore, not all imperfections of ISO 5817 require a fatigue evaluation, e.g., spatter (No. 1.23).

The imperfections of ISO 5817 are limited allowance. Some imperfections are not generally allowed, and for the other imperfections, there are limit information as follows:

- 21 imperfections are allowed for quality level D, C, and B (see Table 4.4);
- Six imperfections are not allowed for quality level D, C, and B and for that there is acceptance limit information (see Table 4.5);
- Five imperfections are not allowed for quality level C and B (see Table 4.6);
- Four imperfections are not allowed for quality level B (see Table 4.7);
- Six imperfections have no acceptance limit information (see Table 4.8).

Table 4.5 Imperfections with no allowance for quality level D, C, and B

Quality group	No. according to ISO 5817	Imperfection designation
Surface imperfections	1.1	Cracks
	1.2	End crater crack
	1.5	Lack of fusion
	1.15	Blowholes
Internal imperfections	2.1	Cracks
	2.11	Copper inclusion

Table 4.6 Imperfections with no allowance for quality level C and B

Quality group	No. according to ISO 5817	Imperfection designation
Surface imperfections	1.6	Insufficient root penetration
	1.13	Overlap
Internal imperfections	2.7	Cavity
	2.8	End crater cavity
	2.12	Lack of fusion

Table 4.7 Imperfections with no allowance for quality level B

Quality group	No. according to ISO 5817	Imperfection designation
Surface imperfections	1.3	Surface pore
	1.4	Open end crater
	1.20	Insufficient throat thickness
Internal imperfections	2.13	Incomplete penetration (lack of penetration)

Table 4.8 Imperfections with no quantitative limit information

Quality group	No. according to ISO 5817	Imperfection designation
Surface imperfections	1.18	Root porosity (only quality level D allowed)
	1.19	Insufficient weld start (only quality level D allowed)
	1.21	Excessive throat thickness (only quality level D allowed)
	1.22	Arc strikes (only quality level D allowed)
	1.23	Sputter (related to level D, C, and B)
Internal imperfections	2.2	Micro-crack (related to level D, C, and B)

4.4 The Relationship Between ISO 5817 and Fatigue Strength for Arc-Welded Steel Structures

The ISO 5817, quality system for welds is frequently referenced worldwide and interpreted as a measurement of weld performance. This standard was initially developed from the old German standard DIN 8563 as a measure of workmanship with respect to fabrication, i.e., as a measure of the skill of the individual performing the welding operation. As such, it has been incorporated into a number of training and education programs for welders and weld inspectors. Numerous studies have shown that the link between the existing weld quality classes and static strength or fatigue performance is not consistent. Some acceptance criteria for some weld features or imperfections are found to have little or no influence on fatigue strength. For features which do influence fatigue strength, the acceptance criteria between quality classes do not result in uniform changes in the fatigue strength. Because this system is so widely used, some comments can be made.

In spite of the fact that ISO 5817 has not been developed with structural performance as a primary criterion, it is often interpreted as reflecting structural performance. For this reason, and because it is widely used internationally, it is worth reviewing the relationship between the standard and current best practice guideline with respect to fatigue assessment. Hobbacher and Kassner [12] have reviewed both the existing IIW Recommendations and experimental data in order to establish the link between ISO 5817 and welds which have fatigue strength consistent with the IIW Recommendations [11].

In Tables 4.9, 4.10, and 4.11, the required ISO 5817 limits of imperfections are presented for load-carrying fillet welds with toe failure (FAT 63) or root failure (FAT 40), and in Tables 4.12, 4.13, and 4.14, the required ISO 5817 limits of

Table 4.9 Required surface imperfection quality group in EN ISO 5817:2006–10 for a fillet weld with weld toe fatigue strength FAT 63 and weld root fatigue strength FAT 40 to meet the IIW Fatigue Recommendations for steel after [12]

Imperfection No. in ISO 5817: 2006	Type of imperfection	Remarks	Minimum required quality group for normal quality welds	Limits of imperfection in the required quality group ISO 5817 wall thickness general $t > 3$ mm
1.1	Crack	(Toe and root crack)	D	Not allowed
1.2	End crater crack	(Toe crack)	D	Not allowed
1.3	Surface pore	max diameter of a single pore [mm] (Toe crack)	D	$d \leq 0.3a$ max 3 mm
1.4	Open end crater	Toe crack	D	$0.2t$ max 2 mm

(continued)

Table 4.9 (continued)

Imperfection No. in ISO 5817: 2006	Type of imperfection	Remarks	Minimum required quality group for normal quality welds	Limits of imperfection in the required quality group ISO 5817 wall thickness general $t > 3$ mm
1.5	Lack of fusion	Fracture mechanics assessment recommended	D	Not allowed
	Micro-lack of fusion		D	Allowed
1.7	Continuous undercut	Depth of undercut (Toe crack)	D	$h \leq 0.2t$ max 1 mm
	Non-continuous undercut	Depth of undercut (Toe crack)	D	$h \leq 0.2t$ max 1.0 mm
1.10	Excessive weld overfill	Height of overfill, soft transition, Overfill in dependence of weld width b (Toe crack)	D	$h \leq 1 + 0.25b$ max 10 mm
1.12	Incorrect weld toe	Weld angle α (Toe crack)	D	≥90°
1.15	Blowhole		D	Not allowed
1.16	Excessive asymmetry	In case of no asymmetry by design (Toe crack)	D	$h \leq 2 + 0.2a$
1.18	Root porosity	Porous solidification of weld root (Root crack)	D	Allowed locally
1.19	Insufficient weld start	To be assessed according to similar imperfections in ISO 5817 (Root crack)	D	Allowed locally
1.20	Insufficient weld throat	Recalculation on net weld throat (Root crack)	D	Short imperfection $h \leq 0.3 + 0.1a$ but max 2
1.21	Excessive weld throat		D	Allowed

(continued)

Table 4.9 (continued)

Imperfection No. in ISO 5817: 2006	Type of imperfection	Remarks	Minimum required quality group for normal quality welds	Limits of imperfection in the required quality group ISO 5817 wall thickness general $t > 3$ mm
1.22	Arc strikes	Allowed if the properties of the base metal are not affected! (Toe crack)	D	Not allowed
1.23	Sputter	Dependent on surface requirement (Toe crack)	D	Not allowed

Table 4.10 Required inner imperfection quality group in EN ISO 5817: 2006–10 for a fillet weld with weld toe fatigue strength FAT 63 and weld root fatigue strength FAT 40 to meet the IIW Fatigue Recommendations for steel after [12]

Imperfection No. in ISO 5817: 2006	Type of imperfection	Remarks	Minimum required quality group for normal quality welds	Limits of imperfection in the required quality group ISO 5817 wall thickness general $t > 3$ mm
2.1	Crack	(Toe and root crack)	D	Not allowed
2.2	Micro-crack	(Toe and root crack)	D	Allowed at a special assessment
2.3	Pore porosity	Percentage of projected area in radiography, biggest pore. For details, see standard	D	Multipass ≤ 5 % single pass ≤ 2.5 % $d \leq 0.4a$ max 5 mm
2.4	Pore nest, clustered porosity	Multipass weld. Percentage of projected area in radiography inclusive all other imperfections, reference length 100 mm, biggest pore	C	≤8 % and $d \leq 0.3a$, $d \leq 3$ mm
2.5	Pore line	Percentage of projected area in radiography, biggest pore. For details, see standard	D	Multipass ≤ 16 % single pass ≤ 8 %, $d \leq 0.4 * a$ max 4 mm

(continued)

Table 4.10 (continued)

Imperfection No. in ISO 5817: 2006	Type of imperfection	Remarks	Minimum required quality group for normal quality welds	Limits of imperfection in the required quality group ISO 5817 wall thickness general $t > 3$ mm
2.6	Wormhole	Length l ≤ a	D	$h \leq 0.4 * a$ max $h \leq 2$ max $l \leq a$
2.7	Cavity	Short imperfection apart from surface	D	Short imperfection allowed, but apart from surface. $h \leq 0.4a$ max 4 mm
2.8	End crater cavity	Dimension h or l, which ever is bigger.	D	h or $l \leq 0.2$ t max 2 mm
2.9	• Solid inclusion • Slag inclusion • Flux inclusion • Oxide inclusion	Length l ≤ a	C	$h \leq 0.3 * a$ max $h = 3$ mm max $l = 50$ mm
2.10	Metallic inclusion except copper	Height of inclusion	D	$h \leq 0.4 * a$ max 4 mm
2.11	Copper inclusion		D	Not allowed
2.12	• Lack of fusion • Flank lack of fusion • Interpass lack of fusion • Root lack of fusion	Short imperfection	C	Not allowed
2.13	Lack of penetration	Short imperfection	C	Not allowed

imperfections are presented for butt welds (FAT 90). These tables provide useful information for design of welded structures. These tables provide a realistic basis for a review of ISO 5817 with the proposal to make the quality levels consistent in terms of fatigue. This direct relation gives the possibility to specify a weld quality for required fatigue strength and vice versa. The possibility to specify the quality levels according to the requirements of fatigue design is of a high economic relevance. As shown in Tables 4.9, 4.10, and 4.11, quality class D would be sufficient

Table 4.11 Required weld geometry imperfections and multiple imperfection quality group in EN ISO 5817:2006-10 for a fillet weld with weld toe fatigue strength FAT 63 and weld root fatigue strength FAT 40 to meet the IIW Fatigue Recommendations for steel after [12]

Imperfection No. in ISO 5817:2006	Type of imperfection	Remarks	Minimum required quality group for normal quality welds	Limits of imperfection in the required quality group ISO 5817 wall thickness general $t > 3$ mm
3.1[a]	Axial misalignment	Linear misalignment at cruciform joints with toe crack and transverse load		$e \leq 0.15t$[b]
3.2	Incorrect root gap for fillet welds	Gap h can be compensated by a thicker fillet weld	D	$h \leq 1 + 0.3a$ max 4 mm
4.1	Multiple imperfections in arbitrary section.	Maximum combined height Σh of imperfections	D	$\Sigma h \leq 0.25a$
4.2	Multiple imperfections in longitudinal direction of weld	Percentage of projected area of imperfections in radiography	C	$\Sigma(h\ l) \leq 8\ \%$

[a]This type of imperfection is not an element of EN ISO 5817:2006-10
[b]The limit of imperfection corresponds to FAT 63 according to [12]

Table 4.12 Required surface imperfection quality group in EN ISO 5817:2006-10 for butt weld with fatigue strength FAT 90 to meet the IIW Fatigue Recommendations for steel after [12]

Imperfection No. in ISO 5817:2006	Type of imperfection	Remarks	Minimum required quality group for normal quality welds	Limits of imperfection in the required quality group ISO 5817 Wall thickness general $t > 3$ mm
1.1	Crack		D (also C, B)	Not allowed
1.2	End crater crack		D (also C, B)	Not allowed
1.3	Surface pore	Max diameter of single pore [mm]	B	Not allowed
1.4	Open end crater		B	Not allowed

(continued)

Table 4.12 (continued)

Imperfection No. in ISO 5817:2006	Type of imperfection	Remarks	Minimum required quality group for normal quality welds	Limits of imperfection in the required quality group ISO 5817 Wall thickness general $t > 3$ mm
1.5	Lack of fusion		D (also C, B)	Not allowed
	Micro-lack of fusion		B	Not allowed
1.6	Insufficient root penetration	Only for single-sided butt welds. Height of missing penetration	B	Not allowed
1.7	Continuous undercut	Depth of undercut (Toe crack)	C (also B)	$h \leq 0.1 * t$ max 0.5 mm
	Non-continuous undercut	Depth of undercut (Toe crack)	C (also B)	$h \leq 0.1 * t$ max 0.5 mm
1.8	Root notch	Depth h of soft notch. Short imperfections	B	$h \leq 0.05 * t$ max 0.5
1.9	Excessive weld overfill	Height of overfill, soft transition, (weld angle > 150°) Overfill in dependence of weld width *b*	B	$h \leq 1 + 0.1 * b$ max 5 mm
1.11	Excessive root overfill	Width *b* of root, soft transition	B	$h \leq 1 + 0.2 * b$ max 3 mm
1.12	Incorrect weld toe	Toe angle α	B	≥150°
1.13	Overlap	Width *b*, *h* short imperfection	C (also B)	Not allowed
1.14	Incomplete filled groove	Soft transition, height *h*, short imperfection	B	$h \leq 0.05 * t$ max 0.5 mm
1.15	Blowhole		D (also C, B)	Not allowed

(continued)

Table 4.12 (continued)

Imperfection No. in ISO 5817:2006	Type of imperfection	Remarks	Minimum required quality group for normal quality welds	Limits of imperfection in the required quality group ISO 5817 Wall thickness general $t > 3$ mm
1.17	Root concavity	Soft transition, short imperfection	B	$h \le 0.05 * t$ max 0.5 mm
1.18	Root porosity	Local occurrence	C (also B)	Not allowed
1.19	Insufficient weld start	To be assessed according to similar imperfections in ISO 5817	C (also B)	Not allowed
1.22	Arc strikes	No effect on base metal	C (also B)	Not allowed
1.23	Sputter	Dependent of surface requirement	D (also C, B)	Not allowed

Table 4.13 Required inner imperfection quality group in EN ISO 5817:2006-10 for a butt weld with fatigue strength FAT 90 to meet the IIW Fatigue Recommendations for steel after [12]

Imperfection No. in ISO 5817:2006	Type of imperfection	Remarks	Minimum required quality group for normal quality welds	Limits of imperfection in the required quality group ISO 5817 wall thickness general $t > 3$ mm
2.1	Crack		D (also C, B)	Not allowed
2.2	Micro-crack		C (also B)	Allowed at a special assessment
2.3	Pore porosity	Percentage of projected area in radiography, largest pore. For details, see standard	C	Multipass ≤ 3 % Single pass ≤ 1.5 % $d \le 0.3 * s$ max 4 mm
2.4	Pore nest, clustered porosity	Multipass weld. Percentage of projected area in radiography inclusive of all other imperfections, reference length 100 mm, biggest pore	B+	≤3 % $d \le 0.2s$ $d \le 2.5$ mm B is not sufficient

(continued)

Table 4.13 (continued)

Imperfection No. in ISO 5817:2006	Type of imperfection	Remarks	Minimum required quality group for normal quality welds	Limits of imperfection in the required quality group ISO 5817 wall thickness general $t > 3$ mm
2.5	Pore line	Percentage of projected area in radiography, biggest pore. For details see standard	B	multipass ≤ 4 % single pass ≤ 2 % $d \leq 0.2 * $ s max 2 mm
2.6	Wormhole	Length $l \leq s$	B+	$h \leq 0.2 * s$ max $h \leq 2$ mm as welded: max $l \leq 2.5$ mm, stress relieved: max $l \leq 20$ mm
2.7	Cavity	Short imperfection apart from surface	C (also B)	Not allowed
2.8	End crater cavity	Dimension h or l, whichever is greater	C (also B)	Not allowed
2.9	• Solid inclusion • Slag inclusion • Flux inclusion • Oxide inclusion	Length l ≤ s	B+	h $\leq 0.2 * s$ max $h = 2$ mm as welded: max $l \leq 2.5$ mm, stress relieved: max $l \leq 20$ mm
2.10	Metallic inclusion except copper	Height of inclusion	D	$h \leq 0.4 * s$ max 4 mm
2.11	Copper inclusion		D (also C, B)	Not allowed
2.12	• Lack of fusion • Flank lack of fusion • Interpass lack of fusion • Root lack of fusion	Short imperfection	C (also B)	Not allowed
2.13	Lack of penetration	Short imperfection, butt weld with full penetration by design	C (also B)	Not allowed

Table 4.14 Required weld geometry imperfections and multiple imperfection quality group in EN ISO 5817:2006-10 for a butt weld with fatigue strength FAT 90 to meet the IIW Fatigue Recommendations for steel after [12]

Imperfection No. in ISO 5817: 2006	Type of imperfection	Remarks	Minimum required quality group for normal quality welds	Limits of imperfection in the required quality group ISO 5817 wall thickness general $t > 3$ mm
3.1	Axial misalignment	Plane plates with transversely stresses butt welds	B	$h \leq 0.1t$ max 3 mm
		Transversely circular welds at cylindrical hollow sections	B+	$h \leq 0.5t$ max $h = 1$ mm
3.x	Angular misalignment	The reduction of fatigue strength depends on highly on restraint conditions. The FAT values are merely a rough guidanc.	Contained in ISO5817:2003 but not in 2006 edition	≤1°
4.1	Multiple imperfections in arbitrary section.	Maximum combined height Σh of imperfections.	B	$\Sigma h \leq 0.2t$
4.2	Multiple imperfections in longitudinal direction of weld	Percentage of projected area of imperfections in radiography.	B+	$\Sigma(h\ l) \leq 3$ % B not sufficient

for most imperfection types in order for a load-carrying fillet weld to achieve fatigue strength consistent with IIW Recommendations. For a few imperfection types, quality class C would be needed. With respect to butt welds, there is much more variation with respect to quality class. For some imperfection types, weld quality class D is sufficient while for other imperfection types even weld quality call B is not sufficient.

In applying the principles as depicted above, a correlation between the quality groups B, C, and D in ISO 5817 can be established for each individual type of imperfection and the corresponding fatigue class FAT for a specified wall thickness (see Table 4.15). This was done for an example of a butt weld at 10 mm wall thickness and a fillet weld at also 10 mm wall thickness and a weld throat of 5 mm. The fatigue class FAT is the stress range $\Delta\sigma$ [MPa] at 2 million cycles and $R = \sigma_{min}/\sigma_{max} = 0.5$ for a survival probability of mean minus two standard deviations.

Table 4.15 Matching of quality groups in ISO 5817:2006-10 and fatigue classes FAT in the IIW Recommendations for steel at 10 mm wall thickness and 5 mm weld throat at fillet welds (excerpt)

No. ISO 5817 2006	No. ISO 6520-1 1998	Type of imperfection	Remarks	Maximum usable fatigue class FAT in assessment by nominal stress method for the different quality groups[b]		
				D	C	B
1 Surface imperfections						
1.6	4021	Insufficient root penetration	Verification of net section!	FAT 40	Not allowed	Not allowed
1.7	5011	Continuous undercut	Butt weld	FAT 71	FAT 90	FAT 90
			Fillet weld (Toe crack)	FAT 63	FAT 80	FAT 80
	5012	Non-continuous undercut	Butt weld	FAT 71	FAT 90	FAT 90
			Fillet weld (Toe crack)	FAT 63	FAT 80	FAT 80
1.13	506	Overlap	(Crevice corrosion to be considered!)	FAT 80	Not allowed	Not allowed
2. Inner imperfections						
2.3	2011	Pore	Butt weld, multipass	FAT 80	FAT 100	FAT 125
	2012	Porosity	Fillet weld, multipass (Root crack)	FAT 40	FAT 40	FAT 40
2.4	2013	Pore net clustered porosity	without a special assessment or at an additional limitation of projected area. Butt weld	FAT 50 ≤ 5 %: FAT 71	FAT 63 ≤ 4 %: FAT 80	FAT 71 ≤ 3 %: FAT 90
			Fillet weld (Root crack)	FAT 40	FAT 40	FAT 40
2.5	2014	Pore line	Butt weld, multipass	FAT 71	FAT 80	FAT 90
			Fillet weld, multipass (Root crack)	FAT 40	FAT 40	FAT 40

(continued)

Table 4.15 (continued)

No. ISO 5817 2006	No. ISO 6520-1 1998	Type of imperfection	Remarks	Maximum usable fatigue class FAT in assessment by nominal stress method for the different quality groups[b]		
				D	C	B
2.9	300 301 302 303	Solid inclusion Slag inclusion Flux inclusion Oxide inclusion	Butt weld (height of inclusion < $1/4 \cdot t$) or at additional limitation of length L (see Chap. 3)	FAT 56 $L \leq 10$ mm: FAT 71	FAT 63 $L \leq 4$ mm: FAT 80	FAT 80 $L \leq 2.5$ mm: FAT 90
			Fillet weld (height of inclusion < $1/4a$), root crack (see Chap. 3)	FAT 40	FAT 40	FAT 40
2.10	304	Metallic inclusion except copper	Butt weld (see Chap. 3)	FAT 100	FAT 100	FAT 125
			Fillet weld (Root crack)	FAT 40	FAT 40	FAT 40
2.11	3042	Copper inclusion	Butt weld	Not allowed	Not allowed	Not allowed
			Fillet weld (Root crack)			
3. Imperfections of weld geometry						
3.1	507	Axial misalignment	Calculative verification recommended, if necessary	FAT 45	FAT 63	FAT 90
(3.2)[a]	508	Angular misalignment	Calculative verification recommended, if necessary	FAT 40	FAT 56	FAT 90

[a]This item is no longer part of ISO 5817:2006, but it was contained in ISO 5817:2003. Nevertheless, this item is relevant for fatigue

[b]Only general remarks can be given for engineering assessment. It may be done by verification of the net section using FAT 40, by the effective notch stress method or by fracture mechanics considerations

In 2013, a revised version of ISO 5817 is published, which contains an informative annex C about the relationship between quality levels and fatigue strength. In this annex, the imperfection limits for quality levels of ISO 5817 are related to FAT 63 and FAT 90 according to the contents in [12]. Furthermore, there are also requirements for high-quality fabrication with the relation to FAT 125. Additionally to the imperfections of the main part of ISO 5817, the weld toe radius (No. 5052 in ISO 6520-1) and angular misalignment (No. 508 in ISO 6520-1) are to some extent included in their relationship to these FAT classes.

References

1. ISO/TS 17845:2004; Welding and allied processes – Designation system for imperfections, 2004
2. ISO 6520-1:2007; Welding and allied processes – Classification of geometric imperfections in metallic materials – Part 1: Fusion welding; July 2007
3. ISO 6520-2:2007; Welding and allied processes – Classification of geometric imperfections in metallic materials – Part 2: Welding with pressure, 2001
4. ISO 5817:2006; Welding – Fusion-welded joints in steel, nickel, titanium and their alloys (beam welding excluded) – Quality levels for imperfections (ISO 5817:2003 +Cor. 1:2006), April 2006
5. ISO 10042:2005; Welding – Arc-welded joints in aluminium and its alloys – Quality levels for imperfections, November 2005
6. ISO 13919-1:1996; Welding – Electron and laser beam welded joints – Guidance on quality levels for imperfections – Part 1: Steel, August 1996
7. ISO 13919-2:2001: Welding – Electron and laser beam welded joints – Guidance on quality levels for imperfections – Part 2: Aluminium and its weldable alloys, September 2001
8. ISO 13920:1996: Welding – General tolerances for welded constructions – Dimensions for length and angles, shape and position, 1996
9. ISO 9013:2002; Thermal cutting - Classification of thermal cuts - Geometrical product specification and quality tolerances, 2002
10. ISO 17658:2002; Welding - Imperfections in oxyfuel flame cuts, laser beam cuts and plasma cuts – Terminology, 2002
11. Hobbacher, A. (Editor): Recommendations for fatigue design of welded joints and components. IIW document XIII-2151-07/XV-1254-07. Welding Research Council New York, WRC-Bulletin 520, 2009
12. Hobbacher. A., Kassner, M.: On Relation between Fatigue Properties of Welded Joints, Quality Criteria and Groups in ISO 5817, Welding in the World, No. 11/12, 2012
13. ISO 12932:2013: Welding – Laser-arc hybrid welding of steels, nickel and nickel alloys – Quality levels for imperfections, October 2013

Chapter 5
Weld Quality Levels for Fatigue Loaded Structures

5.1 Assessment of Defects

The imperfections and their classification into quality groups are mostly done by the guidance of introduced codes. One standard for weld quality is ISO 5817. This standard is an adoption of the old German standard DIN 8563, which was established as a standard for communication between the welders and the inspectors. The classification criterion was the difficulties, the expenses, or the efforts to fabricate or to inspect by NDT. So by the nature, ISO 5817 has limits in direct application to fatigue problems, it is inconsistent with respect to fatigue properties and needs application guidance. Most dedicated design codes specify a general quality level according to ISO 5817 and give additional regulations. In this situation, the IIW fatigue design recommendations have extended the scope of usual fatigue design codes by describing the fatigue properties of joints containing weld imperfections on a scientific basis.

After inspection and detection of a weld imperfection, the first step of the assessment procedure is to determine the type and the effect of the imperfection by categorization as given in Table 5.1. If a weld imperfection cannot be clearly associated to a type or an effect of imperfections as listed here, it is recommended that it is assumed to be crack-like. The interpretation of additive imperfections is that they are adding their impact on fatigue, e.g., an undercut and a small toe radius. Competitive imperfections are not influencing each other and so will compete in being the most critical one, e.g., an inner pore and a small toe radius.

B. Jonsson et al., *IIW Guidelines on Weld Quality in Relationship to Fatigue Strength*, IIW Collection, DOI 10.1007/978-3-319-19198-0_5

Table 5.1 Categorization and assessment procedure for weld imperfections

Effect of imperfection		Type of imperfection	Assessment
Rise of general stress level		Misalignment	Formulae for effective stress concentration
Local notch effect	Additive	Weld shape imperfections, undercut	Tables given
	Competitive	Porosity and inclusions not near the surface	Tables given
Crack-like imperfection		Cracks, lack of fusion, and penetration, all types of imperfections other than given here	Fracture mechanics

5.2 Requirements for a Production Standard Weld Quality

In as-welded joints, the fatigue resistance is given by a so-called FAT class. This is the stress range at 2 million cycles for a certain survival probability (see FAT in nomenclature above). The spacing of the grid of resistance S–N curves corresponds to a factor of $\sqrt[20]{10} = 1.122$ (see Fig. 3.2), and so they are arranged in certain defined steps. The other fatigue resistance values in this document also give the data in the same way for 2 million cycles.

5.2.1 Effect of Toe Geometry

Several assessment procedures do not consider the important effects of toe geometry. These are the nominal stress and the structural hot spot procedures, which reflect the toe geometries of the specimens which have been tested for the establishing of the codes or recommendations. A wide scatter of the experimental results is the consequence. There are two assessment procedures, by which the effects can be covered, that are the effective notch stress method and the fracture mechanics evaluation.

The governing parameters for fatigue properties failing from the weld toe are weld transition angle Θ, the toe radius ρ, the weld throat, and the wall thicknesses of the joined plates (see Fig. 2.1).

Various attempts have been made to derive the fatigue properties directly from the shape of the weld toe transition. For those calculations, three geometrical parameters have been used, such as weld toe radius, weld toe angle, and wall thickness.

The mostly used formulae for the stress raising notch effect of the toe have been developed by Lawrence [1], Ushirokawa [2], Nishida [2], Tsuji [2], and Anthes [3]. When calculating a notch factor K_t, it has to be considered that the transition from K_t to K_f is dependent on the stress gradient in thickness direction and so also on the wall thickness.

Since the weld toe radii (ρ) mainly depend on the welding procedure in shop and are independent from the wall thickness, the ratio of radius to wall thickness (ρ/*t*) varies, which in consequence leads to a dependence of fatigue properties of wall thickness, the so-called thickness effect.

Nominal and structural hot spot stress methods do not consider the geometric parameters of the weld toe. They need an extra compensation for the effect of wall thickness. Notch stress and fracture mechanics include this effect.

The fatigue resistance values for the effective notch stress method (with model radius of, e.g., 1 mm) have been directly derived from recalculation of experimental data, and so the effect of the transition from K_t to K_f is implicitly considered. Using fracture mechanics and crack propagation calculations, the decline of stress in thickness direction reduces the crack growth rate accordingly and thus considers the effect of the stress gradient.

5.2.1.1 Toe Radius in Butt Welds

The effect of the toe radius is directly covered by the effective notch and fracture mechanics method. This effect is not covered in the nominal and structural hot spot stress method, and thus, their effects might be estimated using Tables 5.2 and 5.3.

Table 5.2 Maximal usable factor on fatigue resistance at different wall thickness, *t*, and transition radius, *r*, for butt welds (*r* and *t* in mm)

r\t	t = 6	t = 12	t = 25	t = 50
r = 0.2	1.19	1.03	1.00	0.87
r = 0.3	1.25	1.09	1.00	0.87
r = 0.5	1.33	1.16	1.00	0.87
r = 1	1.45	1.26	1.09	0.95
r = 2	1.58	1.38	1.19	1.04
r = 3	1.66	1.45	1.25	1.09

Table 5.3 Maximal usable FAT levels on fatigue resistance at different wall thickness, *t*, and transition radius, *r*, for butt welds (*r* and *t* in mm), note that FAT values always take the next lower level when computed is in between the steps

r\t	t = 6	t = 12	t = 25	t = 50
r = 0.2	100	90	90	71
r = 0.3	112	90	90	71
r = 0.5	112	100	90	71
r = 1	125	112	90	80
r = 2	140	112	100	90
r = 3	140	125	112	90

The assessment of the toe radius may be done after Nykänen, Marquis, and Björk (IIW doc. XIII-2177-07). The used exponent for the effect of radius ρ was taken as 0.125 and that on wall thickness t as 0.2

$$\Delta\sigma \propto \left(\frac{\rho}{t}\right)^{0.125} \quad \text{and} \quad \Delta\sigma \propto \left(\frac{25}{t}\right)^{0.2}$$

Table 5.2 shows the relative factor on fatigue resistance at different wall thicknesses and transition radii, where the basic FAT value of 90 corresponds to 100 % or a factor 1.00 for a thickness of 25 mm, taken from the thickness effect. The table is applicable for the nominal stress approach, and translated data to FAT are given in Table 5.3. The tables also have assumed a "thinnes" effect although this needs to be verified by tests.

For more details about the thickness effect, see Ref. [35] by I. Lotsberg.

The factors given in Tables 5.2 and 5.3 are theoretical values. The usable fatigue strength may be limited by the effect of various weld imperfections. This applies especially at the thin wall thicknesses (see also Refs. [21, 35]).

5.2.1.2 Toe Radius in Fillet Welds

The effect of the toe radius is directly covered by the effective notch and fracture mechanics method. This effect is not covered in the nominal and structural hot spot stress method and thus should be assessed using Table 5.4. The IIW fatigue resistance is FAT 63, 71, or 80 depending on the type of fillet joint. Table 5.4 shows the relative factor on fatigue resistance at different wall thicknesses and transition radii, where the basic FAT value corresponds to 100 % or a factor 1.00 for a thickness of 25 mm, taken from the thickness effect. The table is applicable for the nominal stress approach, and translated data to a basic FAT 80 is given in Table 5.5. The tables also have assumed a "thinnes" effect although this needs to be verified by tests.

Table 5.4 Maximal usable factor on fatigue resistance at different wall thickness, t, and transition radius, r, for fillet welds (r and t in mm)

r\t	$t = 6$	$t = 12$	$t = 25$	$t = 50$
$r = 0.2$	1.37	1.11	1.00	0.81
$r = 0.3$	1.44	1.17	1.00	0.81
$r = 0.5$	1.53	1.25	1.00	0.81
$r = 1$	1.67	1.36	1.09	0.89
$r = 2$	1.82	1.48	1.19	0.97
$r = 3$	1.92	1.56	1.25	1.02

Table 5.5 Maximal usable FAT levels (using a basic FAT 80 fillet joint) on fatigue resistance at different wall thickness, *t*, and transition radius, *r*, for fillet welds (*r* and *t* in mm), note that FAT values always take the next lower level when computed is in between the steps

r\t	t = 6	t = 12	t = 25	t = 50
r = 0.2	100	80	80	63
r = 0.3	112	90	80	63
r = 0.5	112	100	80	63
r = 1	125	100	80	71
r = 2	140	112	90	71
r = 3	140	125	100	80

The assessment of the toe radius may be done after Nykänen, Marquis, and Björk (IIW doc. XIII-2177-07). The used exponent for the effect of radius ρ was taken as 0.125 and that on wall thickness t as 0.3

$$\Delta\sigma \propto \left(\frac{\rho}{t}\right)^{0.125} \quad \text{and} \quad \Delta\sigma \propto \left(\frac{25}{t}\right)^{0.3}$$

Tables 5.4 and 5.5 show the relative factors on fatigue resistance at different wall thicknesses and transition radii.

The factors given in the Tables 5.4 and 5.5 are theoretical values. The usable fatigue strength may be limited by the effect of various weld imperfections. This is applicable especially for thin wall thicknesses and in relation to the weld width (see also Refs. [21, 35]).

5.2.2 *Effect of Misalignment*

Misalignment in axially loaded joints leads to an increase of stress in the welded joint due to the occurrence of secondary shell bending stresses. The resulting stress is calculated by stress analysis or by using the formulae for the stress magnification factor $\mathbf{k_m}$. Formulae for this magnification factors are given (Table 5.6). It can be easily seen that misalignment is a very important factor in fatigue.

Some allowance for misalignment is already included in the tables of classified structural details (Table 5.6). In particular, the data for transverse butt welds already include a misalignment of up to 10 % of wall thickness dependent on the execution of the weld, which results in an increase of stress up to 30 %. For cruciform joints, a misalignment of up to 15 % of wall thickness is included, which leads to an increase

Table 5.6 Consideration of stress magnification factors due to misalignment

Type of k_m analysis	Nominal stress approach	Structural hot spot, effective notch approach and linear fracture mechanics	
Type of welded joint	k_m already covered in FAT class	k_m already covered in S–N curves	Default value of effective k_m to be considered in stress
Butt joint made in shop in flat position	1.15	1.05	1.10[a]
Other butt joints	1.30	1.05	1.25[a]
Cruciform joints	1.45	1.05	1.40[a]
Fillet welds on one plate surface	1.25	1.05	1.20[b]

[a]But not more than $(1 + 2.5 * e_{max}/t)$, where e_{max} = permissible misalignment and t = wall thickness of loaded plate

[b]But not more than $(1 + 0.2 * t_{ref}/t)$, where t_{ref} = reference wall thickness of fatigue resistance curves

of stress up to 45 %. Only exceeding misalignments need to be considered. The effective stress magnification factor $k_{m,eff}$ becomes

$$k_{m,eff} = \frac{k_{m,calculated}}{k_{m,already\ covered}}$$

For joints containing both linear and angular misalignment, both stress magnification factors should be applied using the formula

$$k_m = 1 + (k_{m,axial} - 1) + (k_{m,angular} - 1)$$

For angular misalignment, there is a straightening effect (see Fig. 5.1).
Table 5.7 gives formulae for k_m for the most frequent cases.

5.2.2.1 Misalignment in Butt Welds

The effects of misalignment may be assessed using the table in Sect. 5.2.2. A certain amount of misalignment is already covered in the catalog of structural details, i.e., for butt joints, its k_m = 1.3 which is equivalent to a misalignment $e < 10$ % of the thickness, t. A possible higher misalignment at smaller wall thicknesses should be checked. For angular misalignment, a table can be established with the help of Fig. 5.1 and Table 5.8. For more results, see Refs. [21, 35].

In the following table, the effect of axial misalignment e is given by a factor to the basic fatigue resistance FAT [MPa] on an as-welded butt weld allowing up to 10 % misalignment, thus already included in the table. Note that the table is applicable for the nominal stress method only.

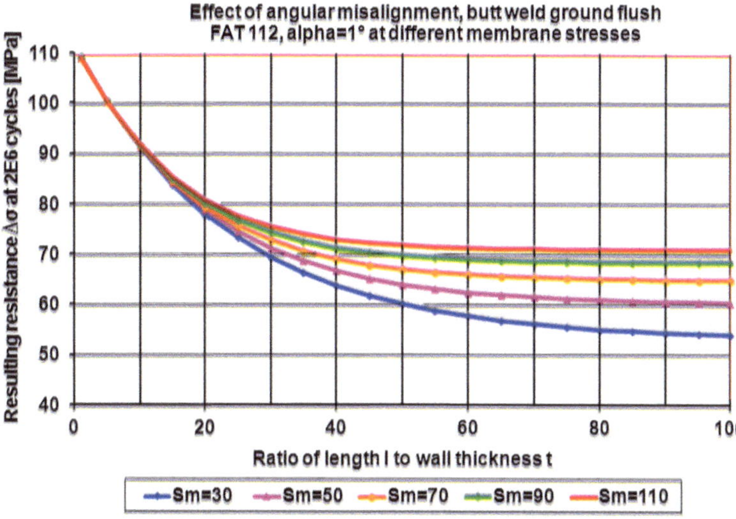

Fig. 5.1 Example of the effect of angular misalignment for tension (Table 5.7 formula #5)

5.2.2.2 Misalignment in Fillet Welds

The effects of misalignment may be assessed using the table in 5.2.2. A certain amount of misalignment is already covered in the catalog of structural details, i.e., for load-carrying fillet joints, its k_m = 1.45 which is equivalent to a misalignment e < 15 % of the thickness, t. A possible higher misalignment at smaller wall thicknesses should be checked. For angular misalignment, a table should be established with the help of Fig. 5.1 and Table 5.9.

In the following table, the effect of axial misalignment e is given by a factor to the basic fatigue resistance FAT on an as-welded cruciform joint, where the catalog of structural details allows a misalignment of up to 15 % of primary plate thickness, thus already included in the table. Note that the table is applicable for the nominal stress method only. Note also that in non-load-carrying joints, a linear misalignment has a minor influence; however, angular misalignment also do (see more data in Refs. [21, 35]).

5.2.3 Effect of Undercut

The basis for the assessment of undercut is the ratio of **u/t**, i.e., depth of undercut to plate thickness. Though undercut is an additive notch, it is already considered to a limited extent in the tables of fatigue resistance of classified structural details. Undercut does not reduce fatigue resistance of welds which are only loaded parallel

Table 5.7 Formulae for assessment of misalignment

No	Type of misalignment	
1	Axial misalignment between flat plates	
	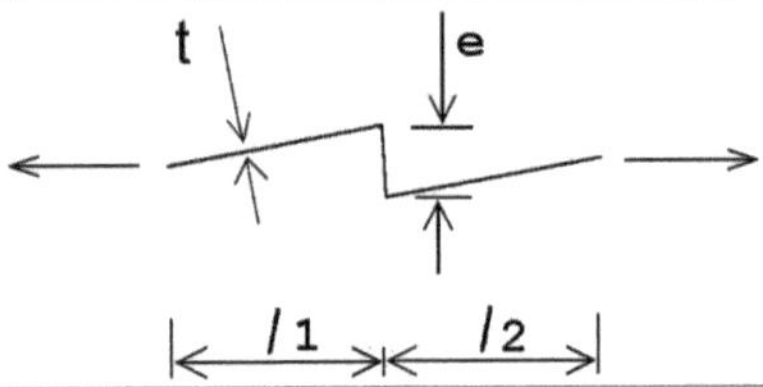	$k_m = 1 + \lambda \cdot \frac{e \cdot l_1}{t \cdot (l_1 + l_2)}$
	λ is dependent on restraint, **λ = 6** for unrestrained joints For remotely loaded joints, assume $\mathbf{l_1 = l_2}$	
2	Axial misalignment between flat plates of differing thickness	
	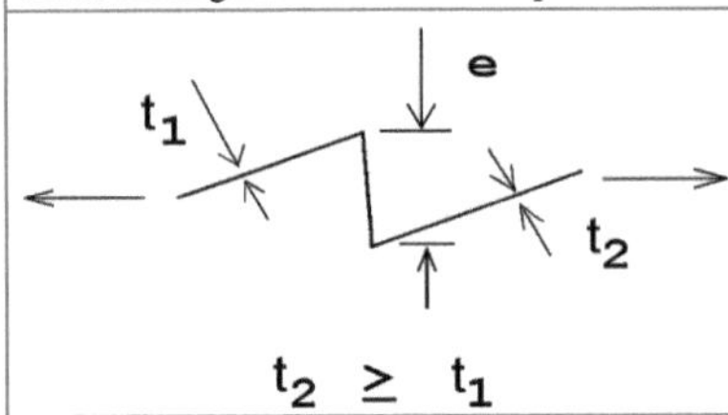	$k_m = 1 + \frac{6e}{t_1} \cdot \frac{t_1^n}{t_1^n + t_2^n}$
	Relates to remotely loaded unrestraint joints The use of **n = 1.5** is supported by tests	
3	Axial misalignment at joints in cylindrical shells with thickness change	
	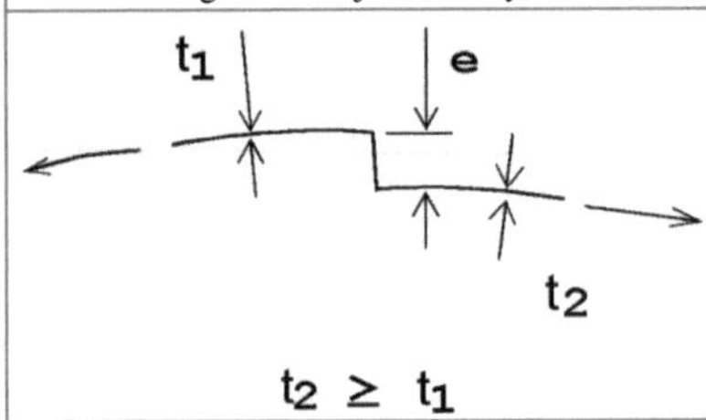	$k_m = 1 + \frac{6e}{t_1 \cdot (1 - \nu^2)} \cdot \frac{t_1^n}{t_1^n + t_2^n}$
	n = 1.5 in circumferential joints and joints in spheres **n = 0.6** for longitudinal joints	
4	Angular misalignment between flat plates	
	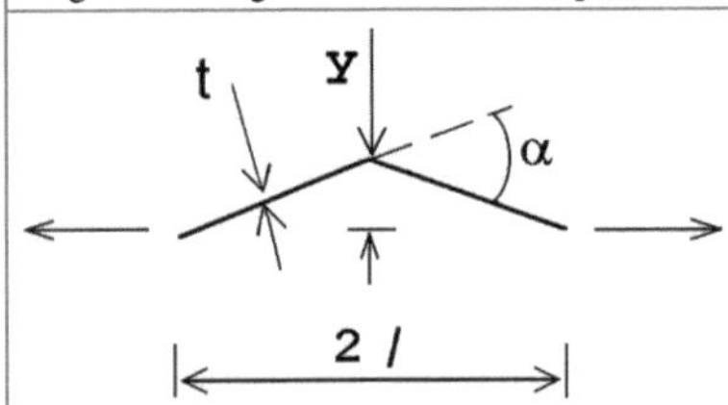	Assuming fixed ends with $\beta = \frac{2l}{t}\sqrt{\frac{3\sigma_m}{E}}$ $k_m = 1 + \frac{3y}{t} \cdot \frac{\tanh(\beta/2)}{\beta/2}$ altern.: $k_m = 1 + \frac{3}{2} \cdot \frac{\alpha \cdot l}{t} \cdot \frac{\tanh(\beta/2)}{\beta/2}$ Assuming pinned ends: $k_m = 1 + \frac{6y}{t} \cdot \frac{\tanh(\beta)}{\beta}$ altern.: $k_m = 1 + \frac{3\alpha \cdot l}{t} \cdot \frac{\tanh(\beta)}{\beta}$
	The **tanh** correction allows for reduction of angular misalignment due to the straightening of the joint under tensile loading. It is always **≤1** and it is conservative to ignore it. σ_m is membrane stress range	

(continued)

Table 5.7 (continued)

No	Type of misalignment	
5	Angular misalignment at longitudinal joints in cylindrical shells	
	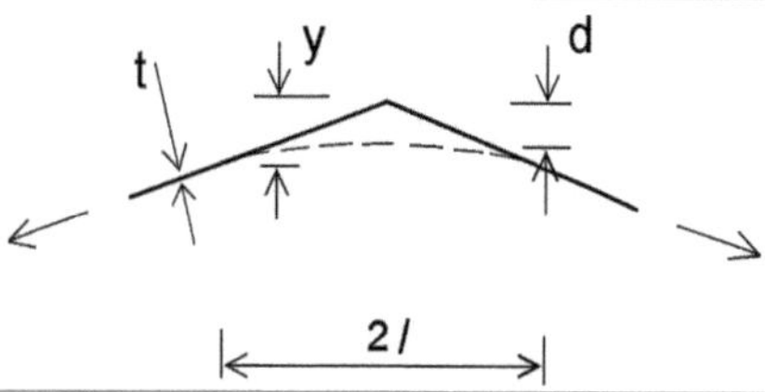	Assuming fixed ends with $\beta = \frac{2l}{t}\sqrt{\frac{3(1-\nu^2)\cdot\sigma_m}{E}}$ $k_m = 1 + \frac{3d}{t(1-\nu^2)} \cdot \frac{\tanh(\beta/2)}{\beta/2}$ assuming pinned ends $k_m = 1 + \frac{6d}{t(1-\nu^2)} \cdot \frac{\tanh(\beta)}{\beta}$
	d is the deviation from the idealized geometry	
6	Ovality in pressurized cylindrical pipes and shells	
	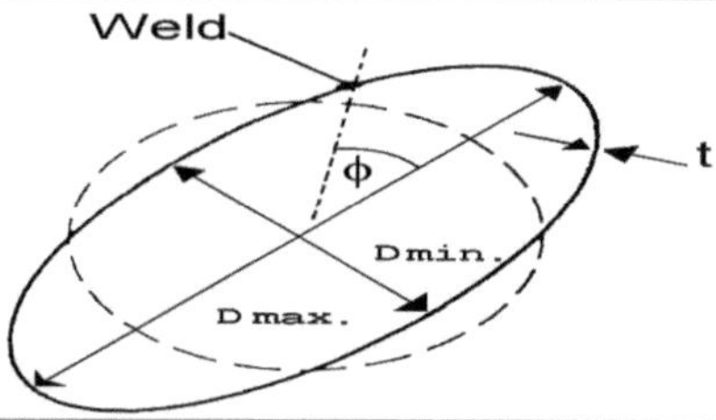	$k_m = 1 + \frac{1.5 \cdot (D_{max} - D_{min}) \cdot \cos(2\Phi)}{t \cdot \left(1 + \frac{0.5 \cdot p_{max} \cdot (1-\nu^2)}{E}\left(\frac{D}{t}\right)^3\right)}$
7	Axial misalignment of cruciform joints (toe cracks)	
	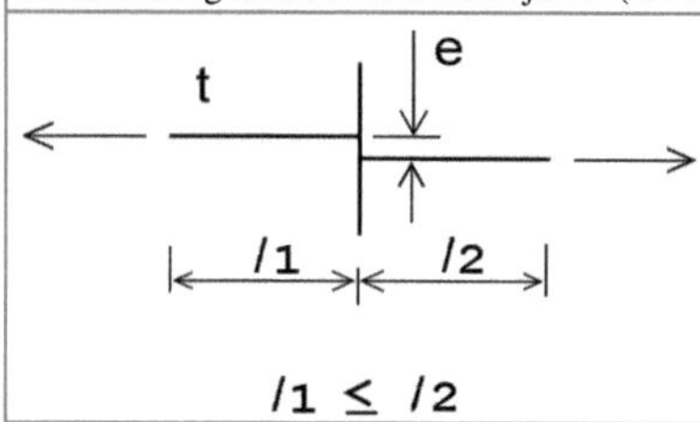	$k_m = 1 + \lambda \cdot \frac{e \cdot l_1}{t \cdot (l_1 + l_2)}$ λ is dependent on restraint
	λ varies from λ = **3** (fully restrained) to λ = **6** (unrestraint). For unrestrained remotely loaded joints, assume: $\mathbf{l_1 = l_2}$ and λ = **6**	
8	Angular misalignment of cruciform joints (toe cracks)	
	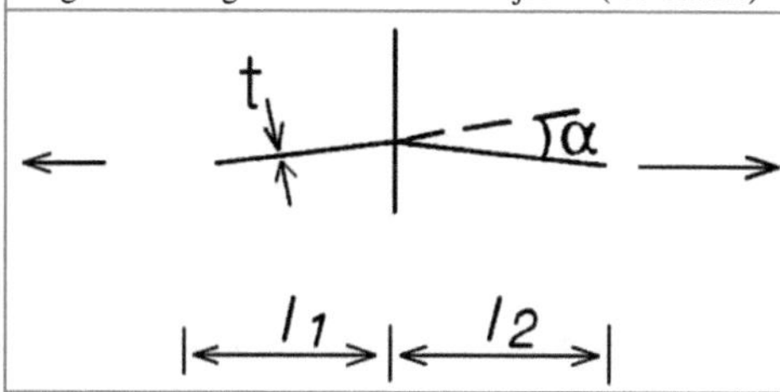	$k_m = 1 + \lambda \cdot \alpha \cdot \frac{l_1 \cdot l_2}{t \cdot (l_1 + l_2)}$ λ is dependent on restraint
	If the in-plane displacement of the transverse plate is restricted, λ varies from λ = 0.02 to λ = **0.04**. If not, λ varies from λ = **3** to λ = **6**	

(continued)

Table 5.7 (continued)

No	Type of misalignment	
9	Axial misalignment in fillet welded cruciform joints (root cracks)	
	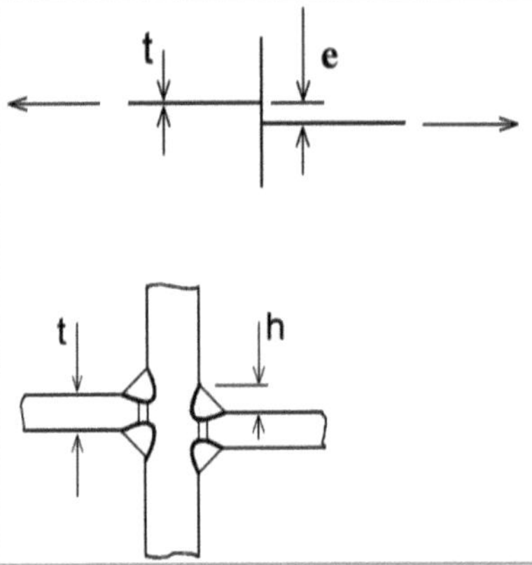	$k_m = 1 + \frac{e}{t+h}$
	k_m refers to the stress range in weld throat	

Table 5.8 Maximal usable factor on fatigue resistance at different wall thicknesses and misalignments for butt welds (*e* and *t* in mm)

e\t	$t = 6$	$t = 12$	$t = 25$	$t = 50$
$e = 0.5$	1.04	1.16	1.23	1.26
$e = 1$	0.87	1.04	1.16	1.23
$e = 2$	0.65	0.87	1.05	1.16
$e = 5$	–	0.58	0.81	1.00
$e = 10$	–	–	0.59	0.81

Table 5.9 Maximal usable factor on fatigue resistance at different wall thicknesses and misalignment for fillet welds (*e* and *t* in mm)

e\t	$t = 6$	$t = 12$	$t = 25$	$t = 50$
$e = 0.5$	1.16	1.29	1.37	1.41
$e = 1$	0.97	1.16	1.29	1.37
$e = 2$	0.73	0.97	1.17	1.29
$e = 5$	–	0.64	0.91	1.12
$e = 10$	–	–	0.66	0.91

to the weld seam. Experimental results and data from the literature lead eventually to the acceptance levels in Table 5.10

5.2.3.1 Undercut in Butt Welds

The effect of undercut can be assessed directly using the effective notch stress or fracture mechanics method. A rapid assessment may be done using Table 5.10 in Sect. 5.2.3.

Table 5.10 Acceptance levels for weld toe undercut in steel

Fatigue class	Allowable undercut u/t	
	Butt welds	Fillet welds
100	0.025	Not applicable
90	0.05	Not applicable
80	0.075	0.05
71	0.10	0.075
63	0.10	0.10
56 and lower	0.10	0.10

Notes
(a) Undercut deeper than 1 mm assessed like a crack
(b) The table is valid for plate thicknesses from 10 to 20 mm

5.2.3.2 Undercut in Fillet Welds

The effect of undercut can be assessed directly using the effective notch stress or fracture mechanics method. A rapid assessment may be done using Table 5.10 in Sect. 5.2.3.

5.2.4 Effect of Cold Laps

When the welding process is not correct, a so-called *cold lap* might be the result. It occurs when the melted weld material does not fully merge with the plate material, leaving a non-fused zone at the weld toe. In a worst case, the cold lap is all along the weld, but sometimes, the cold lap is very local, for instance, when caused by spatter. This is a defect-oriented in parallel with the plate surface, often very small (microscopic), but sometimes bigger for instance when overflow of weld material occurs.

Studies made on this crack-like defect reveal that the growth direction, at least for a weld under tension, quickly will change from being in parallel with the plate at the start to a direction being perpendicular to the plate (see Figs. 5.2 and 5.3).

Studying the crack growth for a line cold lap all along a weld line in a 2D model, one can see that the stress intensity factor (SIF) follows a certain pattern (see Fig. 5.3). As shown, the initial cold lap size has quite a big impact on the SIF value, but after a short growth when the crack has changed direction, the SIF values are approximately the same or having even lower values for bigger cold laps compared to smaller cold laps. The overall result is that the fatigue life is not so sensitive to the starting cold lap size: If there is a cold lap over a certain size (appr. 0.2 mm), then it will quickly turn into a crack perpendicular to the stress direction and lead to failure. The spatter-induced cold lap having a semi-elliptical form ($a/c = 1$) has 2–3 times longer life than the above-studied case in 2D ($a/c = 0$) (see Ref. [16, 17]). Forming rules for cold laps should thus be made assuming line cold laps (conservatively) and using absolute values rather than relative ones. Table 5.11 below

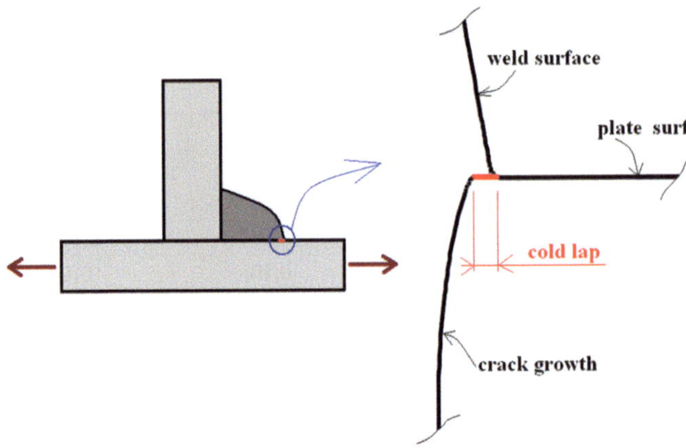

Fig. 5.2 Crack growth from a cold lap

Fig. 5.3 SIFs in cold laps

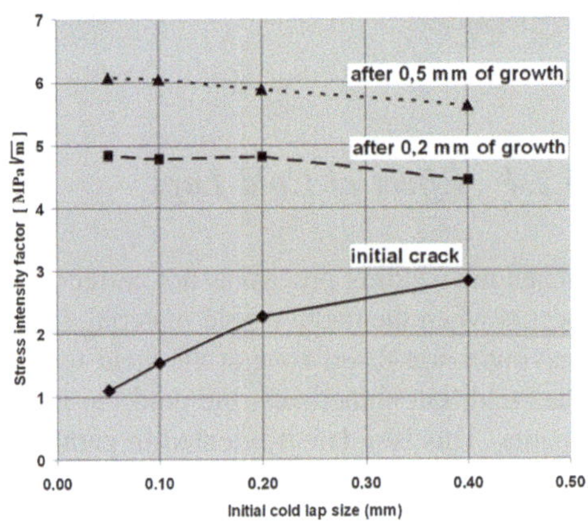

Table 5.11 Acceptance limits for weld toe cold laps in steel

	Allowable cold lap sizes (mm)	
Fatigue class	Butt welds	Fillet welds
63	1.0	1.0
71	1.0	0.1
80	1.0	0.1
90	1.0	Not applicable
100	0.1	Not applicable

tries to give FAT values for such cold laps, compared with Figs. 5.2, 5.3, and 5.4, where analysis of a non-load-carrying fillet weld and a 2-sided welded butt joint has been carried out. Note that a well-done blasting operation after welding probably will prevent the small cold laps (<0.1–0.3 mm) to grow to failure.

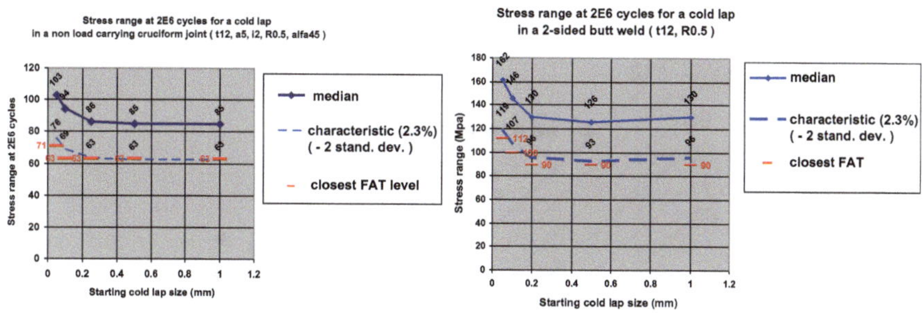

Fig. 5.4 Computed stress ranges for different starting cold lap sizes

5.2.4.1 Cold Laps in Butt Welds

The cold lap is conservatively assumed to be continuous along the fusion line and is described as being in parallel with the ground plate line. The allowable FAT levels are described earlier (see Table 5.11). It is assumed that a blasting operation after welding will prevent a lot of cold laps to develop into failures.

5.2.4.2 Cold Laps in Fillet Welds

The cold lap is conservatively assumed to be continuous along the fusion line and is described as being in parallel with the ground plate line. The allowable FAT levels are described earlier (see Table 5.11). It is assumed that a blasting operation after welding will prevent a lot of cold laps to develop into failures.

5.2.5 *Effect of Inclusions and Porosity*

Embedded volumetric discontinuities, such as porosity and inclusions (see Figs. 5.5 and 5.6), are considered as competitive weld imperfections which can provide alternative sites for fatigue crack initiation than those covered by the fatigue resistance tables of classified details. The difference between the allowable size at as-welded and thermally stress-relieved components is attributed to the effusion of hydrogen in annealed welds [18, 19]. New Japanese investigations suggest that at least at thick-walled structures, higher allowable sizes at as-welded joints could be possible. This was left to future discussions.

Before assessing the imperfections with respect to fatigue, it should be verified that the conditions apply for competitive notches, i.e., that the anticipated sites of crack initiation in the fatigue resistance tables do not coincide with the porosity and inclusions to be assessed and no interaction is expected. It is important to ensure that there is no interaction between multiple weld imperfections, be it from the same

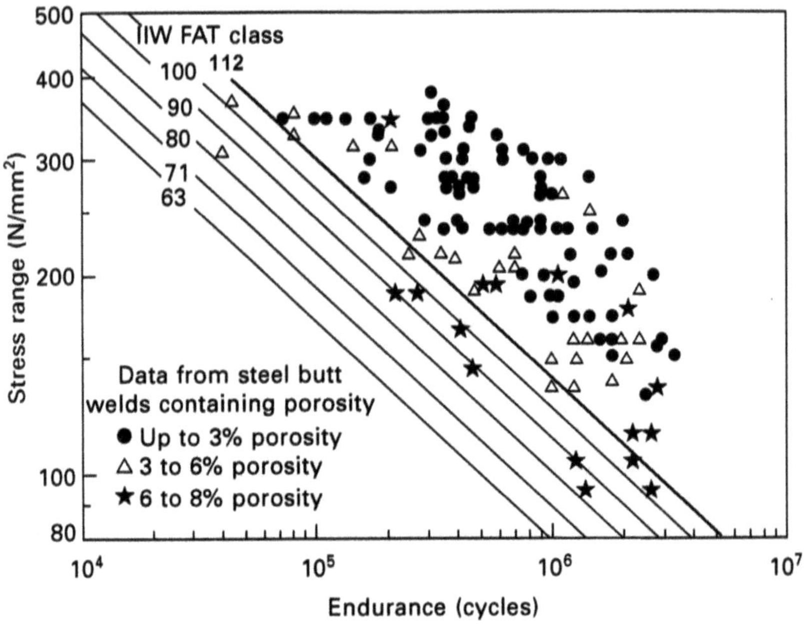

Fig. 5.5 Effect of porosity

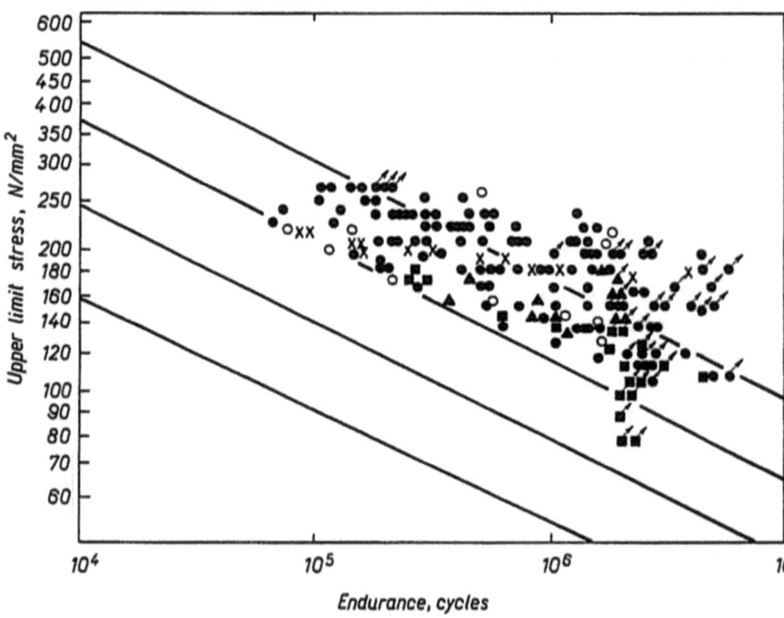

Fig. 5.6 Effect of slag inclusions

Table 5.12 Acceptance levels for porosity and inclusions in welds in steel

Fatigue class	Max. length of an inclusion in mm		Limits of porosity in % of area[a,b]
	As-welded	Stress relieved[c]	
112	–	–	3
100	1.5	7.5	3
90	2.5	19	3
80	4	58	3
71	10	No limit	5
63	35	No limit	5
56 and lower	No limit	No limit	5

[a]Area of radiograph
[b]Max pore diameter or width of inclusion < than 1/4 thickness or 6 mm
[c]Stress relieved by post-weld heat treatment

or different type. Evaluations of fatigue test results containing different types of inclusions and porosity result in Table 5.12.

Surface-breaking pores and blowholes are usually detected by visual inspection and repaired. So no specific recommendations are given here.

5.2.5.1 Inclusions and Porosity in Butt Welds

The effect of inclusions and porosity may be assessed using Table 5.12 in Sect. 5.2.5.

5.2.5.2 Inclusions and Porosity in Fillet Welds

The effect of inclusions and porosity may be assessed using Table 5.12 in Sect. 5.2.5.

5.2.6 *Effect of Cracks and Crack-Like Imperfections*

Planar discontinuities, cracks, or crack-like defects are identified by nondestructive testing and inspection. NDT indications are idealized as elliptical cracks for which the stress intensity factor is calculated. A simplified procedure has been developed which is based on the integration of the crack propagation law from an initial defect size $\mathbf{a_i}$ to defect size of 0.75 % of wall thickness. This cracked component has a lower Wohler S–N curve than initial one. The new fatigue class can be calculated and tabulated in advance. In Tables 5.13, 5.14, and 5.15, the stress ranges at 2×10^6

Table 5.13 Computed stress ranges (Mpa) at 2E6 cycles and characteristic values

Surface cracks at butt weld toes

long surface crack near plate edge, butt welds a/c=0.1

a_i \ t =	3	4	5	6	8	10	12	14	16	20	25	30	35	40	50	100
25.0	0	0	0	0	0	0	0	0	0	0	0	0	0	4	7	17
20.0	0	0	0	0	0	0	0	0	0	0	0	4	6	8	11	20
16.0	0	0	0	0	0	0	0	0	0	0	4	7	9	11	15	23
12.0	0	0	0	0	0	0	0	0	0	6	9	12	14	16	20	27
10.0	0	0	0	0	0	0	0	0	5	9	12	15	18	20	23	29
8.0	0	0	0	0	0	0	4	7	9	13	17	19	22	23	26	32
6.0	0	0	0	0	0	6	9	12	15	18	22	25	26	28	30	35
5.0	0	0	0	0	6	10	13	16	18	22	25	28	29	31	33	38
4.0	0	0	0	5	10	14	18	21	23	26	29	31	33	34	36	40
3.0	0	0	7	11	16	21	24	27	29	31	34	36	37	38	40	43
2.0	5	11	16	20	26	30	32	34	36	38	40	42	43	44	45	48
1.0	22	29	33	36	40	43	45	46	47	49	51	52	52	53	53	54
0.5	41	45	48	50	53	55	57	58	58	59	60	60	60	60	60	59
0.2	61	64	66	68	69	70	70	70	70	70	70	70	69	69	68	64

long surface crack apart from edge, butt welds a/c=0.1

a_i \ t =	3	4	5	6	8	10	12	14	16	20	25	30	35	40	50	100
25.0	0	0	0	0	0	0	0	0	0	0	0	0	0	8	13	23
20.0	0	0	0	0	0	0	0	0	0	0	0	7	11	13	17	26
16.0	0	0	0	0	0	0	0	0	0	0	9	12	15	18	21	29
12.0	0	0	0	0	0	0	0	0	0	11	15	18	21	23	26	33
10.0	0	0	0	0	0	0	0	0	10	15	19	22	25	27	29	36
8.0	0	0	0	0	0	0	8	12	15	20	24	27	29	31	33	39
6.0	0	0	0	0	0	12	16	19	22	26	30	32	34	35	37	43
5.0	0	0	0	0	11	17	20	24	26	30	33	35	37	38	40	45
4.0	0	0	0	9	17	22	26	29	31	34	37	39	41	42	44	48
3.0	0	0	13	18	25	29	32	35	37	40	42	44	45	46	48	51
2.0	11	19	25	29	35	38	41	43	45	47	49	50	51	52	53	55
1.0	33	39	43	46	50	53	54	56	57	59	60	61	61	61	62	61
0.5	52	56	59	61	64	66	67	68	68	69	69	69	69	69	68	66
0.2	74	77	78	79	80	81	81	80	80	80	79	78	77	76	75	70

short surface crack apart from edge, butt welds a/c=0.5

a_i \ t =	3	4	5	6	8	10	12	14	16	20	25	30	35	40	50	100
25.0	0	0	0	0	0	0	0	0	0	0	0	0	0	17	23	36
20.0	0	0	0	0	0	0	0	0	0	0	0	15	21	24	29	40
16.0	0	0	0	0	0	0	0	0	0	0	18	23	27	30	34	43
12.0	0	0	0	0	0	0	0	0	0	21	27	32	35	37	41	47
10.0	0	0	0	0	0	0	0	0	20	27	33	37	39	41	44	50
8.0	0	0	0	0	0	0	18	24	28	34	39	42	44	46	48	52
6.0	0	0	0	0	0	23	30	34	37	42	46	48	50	51	53	56
5.0	0	0	0	0	22	31	36	39	42	47	50	52	53	54	56	57
4.0	0	0	0	20	32	38	43	46	48	52	54	56	57	58	59	60
3.0	0	0	26	33	42	47	51	53	55	58	59	61	61	62	62	62
2.0	22	36	43	48	54	58	60	62	63	65	66	67	67	67	67	65
1.0	54	61	65	68	71	73	74	74	75	75	75	75	74	74	73	69
0.5	76	80	82	83	84	84	84	84	84	83	82	81	80	79	77	71
0.2	98	98	98	98	97	95	94	93	92	90	88	86	85	83	81	74

cycles corresponding to the definition of the fatigue classes (FAT) of classified structural details are shown. The tables have been calculated using the correction functions and the weld joint local geometry correction given in references [21] and [24].

Table 5.14 Computed stress ranges (Mpa) at 2E6 cycles and characteristic values

Embedded cracks

a_i	embedded long crack near plate edge a/c=0.1															
25.0	0	0	0	0	0	0	0	0	0	0	0	0	0	4	7	17
20.0	0	0	0	0	0	0	0	0	0	0	0	3	5	7	11	20
16.0	0	0	0	0	0	0	0	0	0	0	4	6	9	11	14	24
12.0	0	0	0	0	0	0	0	0	0	5	8	11	14	16	19	28
10.0	0	0	0	0	0	0	0	0	4	8	12	15	17	19	23	31
8.0	0	0	0	0	0	0	3	6	8	12	16	19	22	24	27	35
6.0	0	0	0	0	0	5	9	12	14	18	22	25	27	29	32	40
5.0	0	0	0	0	5	9	12	15	18	22	26	28	31	32	35	43
4.0	0	0	0	4	9	14	17	20	23	26	30	33	35	37	39	47
3.0	0	0	6	10	16	20	24	27	29	32	36	38	40	42	45	52
2.0	4	10	15	19	25	30	33	36	38	41	44	46	48	50	52	59
1.0	22	29	33	37	42	46	49	51	53	56	59	61	63	64	67	73
0.5	42	47	52	55	60	63	66	68	69	72	75	77	79	80	82	88
0.2	68	73	77	80	84	87	90	92	93	96	98	100	101	103	105	110
t =	3	4	5	6	8	10	12	14	16	20	25	30	35	40	50	100

a_i	embedded long crack apart from plate edge a/c=0.1															
25.0	0	0	0	0	0	0	0	0	0	0	0	0	0	13	19	30
20.0	0	0	0	0	0	0	0	0	0	0	0	12	17	20	24	33
16.0	0	0	0	0	0	0	0	0	0	0	14	19	22	25	29	37
12.0	0	0	0	0	0	0	0	0	0	17	22	26	29	31	34	41
10.0	0	0	0	0	0	0	0	0	16	22	27	30	33	35	37	44
8.0	0	0	0	0	0	0	14	19	23	28	32	35	37	39	41	48
6.0	0	0	0	0	0	19	24	28	31	35	38	41	42	44	46	53
5.0	0	0	0	0	18	25	29	33	35	39	42	44	46	47	49	56
4.0	0	0	0	15	26	31	35	38	40	43	46	48	50	51	54	59
3.0	0	0	21	27	35	39	42	45	46	49	52	54	56	57	59	64
2.0	17	29	35	40	45	49	51	53	55	58	60	62	64	65	67	71
1.0	44	51	55	58	62	65	67	69	70	73	75	77	78	79	80	84
0.5	65	69	73	75	79	82	84	85	86	88	90	91	92	93	94	97
0.2	91	95	98	100	103	105	106	107	108	110	111	112	112	113	114	117
t =	3	4	5	6	8	10	12	14	16	20	25	30	35	40	50	100

a_i	embedded short crack apart from plate edge a/c=0.5															
25.0	0	0	0	0	0	0	0	0	0	0	0	0	0	20	27	41
20.0	0	0	0	0	0	0	0	0	0	0	0	17	24	28	34	46
16.0	0	0	0	0	0	0	0	0	0	0	20	27	32	35	40	50
12.0	0	0	0	0	0	0	0	0	0	24	32	37	41	43	47	55
10.0	0	0	0	0	0	0	0	0	23	32	38	42	45	48	51	58
8.0	0	0	0	0	0	0	20	28	33	40	45	48	51	53	56	62
6.0	0	0	0	0	0	27	35	40	43	48	53	56	58	59	62	67
5.0	0	0	0	0	26	36	42	46	49	54	57	60	62	63	66	71
4.0	0	0	0	23	37	44	49	53	56	60	63	65	67	68	70	75
3.0	0	0	31	39	49	54	58	61	64	67	70	71	73	74	76	80
2.0	26	42	50	55	62	67	70	72	74	76	79	80	81	82	84	87
1.0	62	70	75	78	83	86	88	89	91	92	94	95	96	97	98	100
0.5	88	93	96	99	102	104	105	106	107	108	110	110	111	112	112	115
0.2	118	121	123	124	126	128	129	129	130	131	132	133	133	134	135	137
t =	3	4	5	6	8	10	12	14	16	20	25	30	35	40	50	100

The real problem in nondestructive testing is the determination of the dimensions of a crack or a crack-like imperfection. These dimensions are needed for calculative assessment. It is hoped that in the near future, imaging procedures will be available, by which these dimensions are directly visible. This point is important, because all fracture mechanics procedures are sensitive to the location and dimensions of the initial flaw.

Table 5.15 Computed stress ranges (Mpa) at 2E6 cycles and characteristic values

Surface cracks at fillet weld toes

a_i	long surface crack near plate edge, fillet welds a/c=0.1															
25.0	0	0	0	0	0	0	0	0	0	0	0	0	0	4	7	16
20.0	0	0	0	0	0	0	0	0	0	0	0	4	6	8	11	19
16.0	0	0	0	0	0	0	0	0	0	0	4	7	9	11	15	22
12.0	0	0	0	0	0	0	0	0	0	6	9	12	14	16	19	25
10.0	0	0	0	0	0	0	0	0	5	9	12	15	17	19	22	27
8.0	0	0	0	0	0	0	4	7	9	13	16	19	21	22	25	30
6.0	0	0	0	0	0	6	9	12	15	18	21	23	25	26	28	33
5.0	0	0	0	0	6	10	13	16	18	21	24	26	28	29	31	35
4.0	0	0	0	5	10	14	18	20	22	25	28	29	31	32	33	37
3.0	0	0	7	11	16	20	23	25	27	30	32	33	34	35	37	39
2.0	5	11	16	20	25	28	31	32	34	36	37	39	40	40	41	43
1.0	22	28	32	34	38	40	42	43	44	45	46	47	48	48	48	48
0.5	38	42	45	47	49	51	52	53	53	54	54	54	54	54	54	52
0.2	57	59	61	61	63	63	63	63	63	63	63	62	61	61	60	56
t =	3	4	5	6	8	10	12	14	16	20	25	30	35	40	50	100

a_i	long surface crack apart from edge, fillet welds a/c=0.1															
25.0	0	0	0	0	0	0	0	0	0	0	0	0	0	8	13	22
20.0	0	0	0	0	0	0	0	0	0	0	0	7	11	13	17	25
16.0	0	0	0	0	0	0	0	0	0	0	9	12	15	18	21	28
12.0	0	0	0	0	0	0	0	0	0	11	15	18	21	23	26	32
10.0	0	0	0	0	0	0	0	0	10	15	19	22	24	26	28	34
8.0	0	0	0	0	0	0	8	12	15	20	24	26	28	29	32	37
6.0	0	0	0	0	0	12	16	19	22	26	29	31	33	34	36	40
5.0	0	0	0	0	11	17	20	24	26	29	32	34	35	36	38	42
4.0	0	0	0	9	17	22	26	28	30	33	36	37	39	40	41	44
3.0	0	0	13	18	25	29	32	34	36	38	40	42	43	44	45	47
2.0	11	19	25	29	34	37	39	41	42	44	46	47	48	49	50	51
1.0	32	38	42	44	48	50	52	53	54	55	56	57	57	57	57	56
0.5	50	53	56	58	60	62	63	63	64	64	64	64	63	63	62	59
0.2	70	72	73	74	75	75	74	74	74	73	72	71	70	69	67	62
t =	3	4	5	6	8	10	12	14	16	20	25	30	35	40	50	100

a_i	short surface crack apart from edge, fillet welds a/c=.5															
25.0	0	0	0	0	0	0	0	0	0	0	0	0	0	17	23	35
20.0	0	0	0	0	0	0	0	0	0	0	0	15	21	24	29	38
16.0	0	0	0	0	0	0	0	0	0	0	18	23	27	30	34	42
12.0	0	0	0	0	0	0	0	0	0	21	27	32	35	37	40	45
10.0	0	0	0	0	0	0	0	0	20	27	33	36	39	41	43	47
8.0	0	0	0	0	0	0	18	24	28	34	39	41	43	45	47	49
6.0	0	0	0	0	0	23	30	34	37	42	45	47	48	49	51	52
5.0	0	0	0	0	22	31	36	39	42	46	48	50	51	52	53	53
4.0	0	0	0	20	32	38	42	45	47	50	52	54	54	55	55	55
3.0	0	0	26	33	42	47	50	52	53	55	57	58	58	58	58	57
2.0	22	36	43	48	53	56	58	60	61	62	62	62	62	62	62	59
1.0	53	60	63	66	68	69	70	70	70	70	69	69	68	67	66	62
0.5	74	76	78	78	79	78	78	77	77	76	74	73	72	71	69	64
0.2	92	91	91	90	88	86	85	84	83	81	79	77	75	74	72	65
t =	3	4	5	6	8	10	12	14	16	20	25	30	35	40	50	100

5.2.6.1 Crack-Like Imperfections in Butt Welds

A rapid and conservative assessment may be done using Table 5.13. Different crack geometries have been used to calculate the fatigue life of the joint. The table gives the fatigue resistance at 2 million cycles in MPa for different initial crack

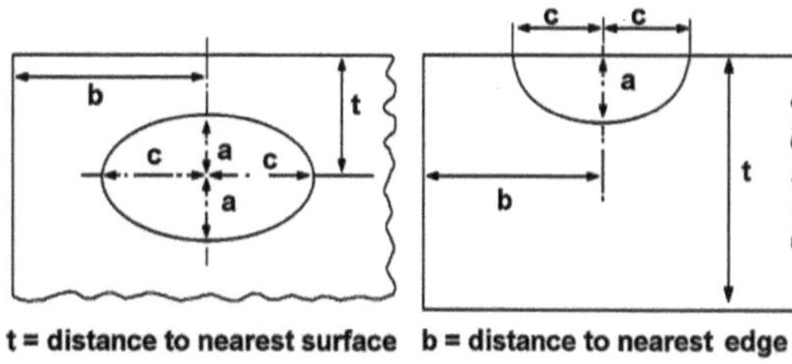

Fig. 5.7 Dimensions of crack

dimensions a_i and different wall thicknesses t. The dimensions of the crack are derived from the circumscribing ellipse (see Fig. 5.7).

5.2.6.2 Crack-Like Imperfections in Fillet Welds

See Table 5.15.

5.3 Design of Experiments (DOE) Using Simulation

Using the effective notch method, many of the above-listed effects can be modeled and one way to show the impact on fatigue is to use design of experiments (DoE) [33]. In such an approach, the physical experiments normally used are replaced by simulations, where the parameters are assigned two levels: one high and one low, preferably on each side of normal values. As an example, if normally a thickness of 10 mm is used, then high level could be 12 and low level could be 8. Or as another example, if normally a throat size of 5 mm is used, then high level could be 6 and low level could be 4.

5.3.1 Parameters Using the Effective Notch Method on Butt Welds

Studying a 1-sided and a (symmetric) 2-sided butt weld where thickness, penetration, angle, undercut, and weld toe radius are given two levels (high and low) and computing the effect of these on the stresses, the result shown in Figs. 5.8 and 5.9 can be found.

As shown, the most important parameters concerning the weld outside are the undercut and the weld toe radius. Other parameters, penetration, thickness, and angle, play a smaller role under the circumstances modeled. Note that the critical point for these cases is the weld root side whenever there is not a full penetration.

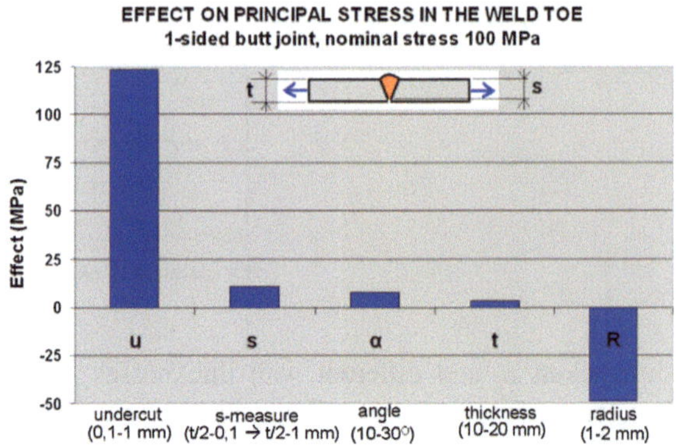

Fig. 5.8 Effects 1-sided butt joint

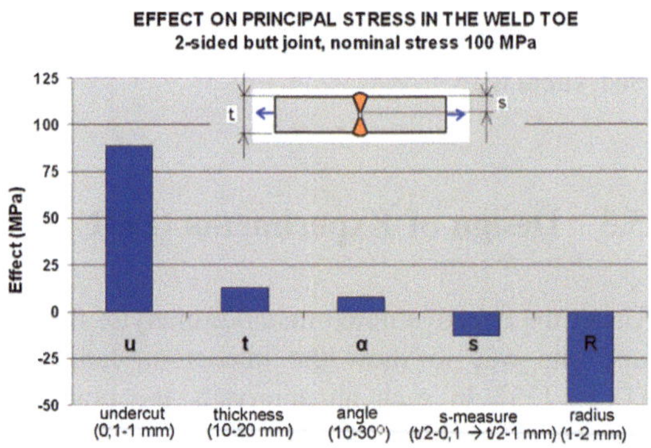

Fig. 5.9 Effects 2-sided butt joint

5.3.2 Parameters Using the Effective Notch Method on Fillet Welds

Studying a load-carrying (LC) and non-load-carrying (non-LC) fillet in a cruciform joint weld where thickness, penetration, angle, undercut, and weld toe radius are given two levels (high and low) and computing the effect of these on the stresses, the result shown in Fig. 5.10 can be found.

First observation is that the influence from the parameters concerning the weld outside is much higher on a LC-joint compared to a non-LC-joint. Next is that the most important parameters are the undercut and the weld toe radius, much the same as for a butt weld. Other parameters, penetration, thickness, angle, misalignment, and angle, play a medium or smaller role under the circumstances modeled. Note that the critical point for the LC-case is normally the weld root side whenever there is not a full penetration.

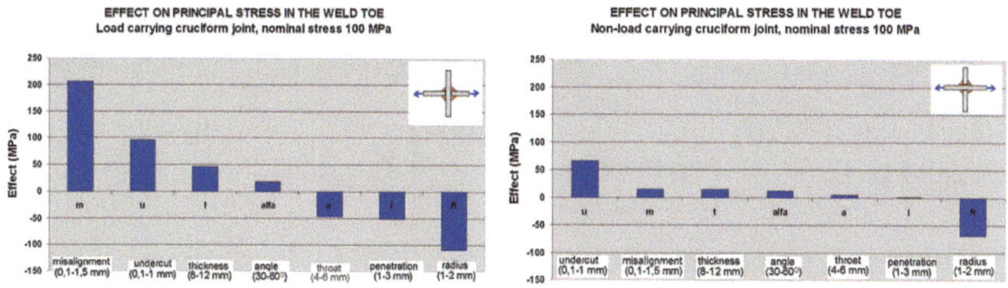

Fig. 5.10 Stress effects from parameters on a LC and non-LC cruciform joint

5.4 Fatigue Design of High-Quality Welds

The term "high quality" is used for welds with a lower level of imperfections as usually accepted. Further on, it is used for welds which are produced under a higher level of control during assembly, accuracy of fit, welding, and inspection of the welded component. Thus, the scatter of fatigue strength can be reduced, and higher stresses might be allowable. In addition, the fatigue strength may be verified by fatigue testing of the component.

The level of control and inspection is laid down in several standards as, e.g., in ISO 3834: quality requirements for fusion welding of metallic material. Here, three levels are specified. A further approach is EN 1090-2009: execution of steel structures and aluminum structures. Here, our execution classes EXC1 to EXC4 are specified and related to the quality groups D to B+ of ISO 5817. The questions of consistence in terms of fatigue in ISO 5817 are not addressed and are still open. One industrial standard used within Volvo CE has been developed, where acceptance limits are formulated to relate to fatigue (see Ref. [29]), here one quality level is aiming to reflect the fatigue described within IIW Recommendations and there are further one higher and one lower quality level. Apart from stating a connection to fatigue, this industrial standard (STD 181-0004) has at least two main differences compared to ISO 5817: First is that focus is put on the weld toe transition area and thus requirements on the toe radius; and second is that a requirement is defined for the penetration as a measure on the drawing (see Sect. 6.2). These points support the designer to establish an appropriate weld quality level on the drawing. Also, it makes it possible to develop adapted weld processes in workshop to match the different weld designations on the drawing (see more in Ref. [34]).

All benefits of the high-quality welds vanish if significant imperfections are present. In these cases the tables given above in the chapter apply.

5.4.1 *Effect of Improvement Methods*

The fatigue strength can be improved by different methods of post-weld treatments. The benign effect of some improvement methods is already known, and it is already

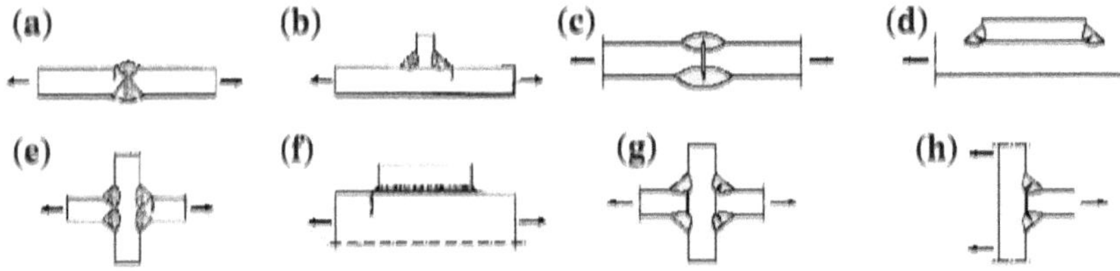

Fig. 5.11 Suitable for improvement (**a**)–(**d**), and not suitable for improvement (**e**)–(**h**)

applied at large series productions. In this case, the fatigue strength has to be verified by test. The new update of the IIW Recommendations has a real novelty, which is a calculative verification of fatigue properties at post-weld treatments. Only factors are given, without a consideration to a possibly flatter slope of the Wohler S–N curves (Fig. 5.11).

The practically applied methods can be divided into two groups: improvement of shape and improvement of residual stress conditions. The IIW Recommendations specify the improvement of the weld toe by burr grinding, by TIG dressing, and by hammer and needle peening. It has to be borne in mind that only such welds can be improved, at which the possible crack at the weld toe is governing. It must be always verified if not another spot of a possible crack initiation could become dominant and governing for the fatigue assessment. This is especially the case at unwelded root gaps or faces, at embedded imperfections, and in cases where the direction of loading is parallel to the notch, e.g., in longitudinally loaded welds seams.

Recently made research has also looked at the so-called HFMI post-treatment (high-frequency mechanical improvement) (see [31]). Here, the toe area is treated imposing residual stresses, which improves fatigue properties, and even a beneficial effect from the material yield limit can be utilized.

5.4.2 *Improvement of Shape of Weld Toe*

The shape improvement methods considered in the IIW Recommendations are grinding of the toe and TIG dressing of the toe. The smoothening of the weld toe transition results in a reduction of the notch effect and thus improves the fatigue properties. The improvement is given by a factor in terms of stress. For quality control in shop, a data sheet has been developed equivalent to weld procedure specification (WPS) sheet.

A guidance for improvement of welds and the benefit from improvement in terms of fatigue are given in Ref. [20]. If even higher benefits from improvement are claimed, that has to be verified by tests. An adequate production quality insurance system should be established in order to ensure that the product quality is at least that of the test.

5.4.3 *Improvement by Compressive Residual Stress*

Hammer peening, needle peening, and high-frequency mechanical improvement (HFMI) (see Refs. [20, 31, 32]) introduce a residual compressive stress which is beneficial for the fatigue properties. Some requirements in loading have to be met at the application of the method. There is a limitation in compressive load stresses in order to avoid an overstressing in compression, which after unloading could relax the residual compressive stress, which was introduced by the improvement procedure.

References

References for Toe Geometry

1. Lawrence F.V., Ho N.J., and Mazumdar P.K.: Predicting fatigue resistance of welds. Ann. Rev. of Material Science, 1981, 11, 401-425.
2. Iida K., and Uemura T.: Stress concentration factor formulas, widely used in Japan. IIW doc. XIII-1530-94. (contains: Ushirokawa, Nishida, Tsuji)
3. Anthes R.J., Köttgen V.B. and Seeger T.: Kerbformzahlen von Stumpfstößen und Doppel-T-Stößen (Notch factors of butt welds and cruciform joints) Schweissen und Schneiden, 1993, 45(12), 685-688
4. Bowness D. and Lee M.M.: Weld toe magnification factors for semi-elliptical cracks in T-butt joints. Int. J. Fatigue, 2000, 22(5), 369-387.
5. Hobbacher A.: Stress intensity factors of welded joints. Engng. Fracture Mechanics 1993, 46 (29), 173-182.
6. Shen G., Plumtree A. and Glinka. G.: Weight function for the surface point of semi-elliptical surface crack in a finite thickness plate. Engineering Fracture Mechanics 40 (1991) pp 167-176
7. Hall M.S., Topp D.A. and Dover W.D.: Parametric equations for stress intensity factors in weldments. Project Report TSC/MSH/0244, Technical Software Consultants Ltd., Milton Keynes, U.K. 1990, published in: C.C. Mohanan: Early Fatigue Crack Growth at Welds. Computational Mechanics Publications, Southampton UK 1995
8. Nykänen T., Marquis G. and Björk T.: Simplified assessment of weld quality for fatigue loaded cruciform joints. IIW doc. XIII-2177-07
9. Huther I., Primot L., Lieurade H.P., Janosch J.J., Colchen D. and Debiez S.: Weld quality and the cyclic fatigue strength of steel welded joints. IIW doc. XIII-1563-94
10. Karlsson N. and Lenander P.H.: Analysisi of fatigue life in two weld class systems. Master Thesis, Dept. of Mach. Eng., Linköping University, Linköping Sweden 2005
11. Marquis G., Björk T. and Samuelsson J.: Toward a quality system for fatigue loaded complex structures. IIW doc. XIII-2103-06

References for Misalignment

12. Berge S. and Myhre H.:Fatigue strength of misaligned cruciform and butt welds. IIW doc. XIII-863-77 (Norwegian Maritime Research, vol 5(1977) no. 1
13. Zeman, J.: Aufdachung an Längsnähten zylindrischer Schüsse (Roofing at longitudinal welded joints in pressured cylinders). Technische Überwachung 34 (1993), Nr. 7/8, S. 292/295

References for Undercut

14. Petershagen H.: The influence of undercut on the fatigue strength of welds, a literature survey. Welding in the World, vol 28(1990) no. 7/8, pp 114-125.(IIW doc. XIII-1120-80)
15. Spadae J.R. and Frank K.H.: Fatigue strength of fillet welded transverse stiffeners with undercuts. Report FHWA/TX-05/0-4178-1, Univ. Austin TX USA

References for Cold Laps

16. Residual stress analysis and fatigue assessment of welded steel structures Dr thesis in Lightweight structures, KTH, Stockholm, Sweden 2008 By Zuheir Barsoum, TRITA-AVE 20008:11, ISSN 1651-7660
17. Development of weld quality criteria based on fatigue performance Paper published in vol. 55 of 'Welding in the World', no 11/12 By Bertil Jonsson, Jack Samuelsson, Gary Marquis

References Porosity

18. Harrison J.D.: The basis for a proposed acceptance standard for welded defects: Part I: Porosity. Part II: Slag inclusions. IIW doc. XIII-817-77
19. Miki Ch., Nishikawa K., Takahashi M. and Konushi T. : Effect of embedded defects of horizontal transverse butt welded joints and settings of requested acceptable quality level. IIW doc. XIII.1954-02

Reference Improvement

20. Haagensen P.J. and Maddox S.J.: IIW Recommendations for weld toe improvement by grinding,TIG dressing and hammer peening for steel and aluminium structures.IIW doc. XIII-1815-00 (rev. 24 Feb. 2006)

References, Others

21. Hobbacher A. et al.: Fatigue design of welded joints and components. Abington Publ., Abington Cambridge UK 1996, ISBN 1 85573 315 3, updated in IIW document XIII-196503/XV-1127-03
22. ISO 6520:1982 (EN 26520:1982), Weld irregularities
23. ISO 5817:2006-10, Quality levels for imperfections
24. British Standard BS 7910:2004: Guide for methods for assessing the acceptability of flaws in metallic structures
25. Petershagen H.: The influence of undercut on the fatigue strength of welds - a literature survey. IIW doc. XIII-1313-89
26. Harrison J.D.: The basis for a proposed acceptance standard for welded defects: Part I: Porosity. Part II: Slag inclusions. IIW doc. XIII-817-77
27. Ogle M. H.: Production Weld Quality Standards for Steel and Aluminium Structures. Welding in the World 29(1991), Nr. 11/12, S. 341-362
28. German Welding Society: DVS 705: Empfehlungen zur Auswahl der Bewertungsgruppen nach ISO 5817 (Recommendations for selection of quality level according to ISO 5817

29. Jonsson B.: Revision of Volvo's weld quality system. IIW doc. XIII-WG4-102-08
30. Karlsson N and Lenander P-H.: Analysis of a weld class system. Dept. of Mech. Eng. University of Linköping Sweden, 2005.
31. Gary B. Marquis et.al., Fatigue Strength Improvement of Steel Structures by HFMI: Proposed Fatigue Assessment Guidelines, Paper: IIW- XIII-2452r1-13
32. Gary Marquis et. Al., Fatigue Strength Improvement of Steel Structures by HFMI: Proposed Procedures and Quality Assurance Guidelines, Paper: IIW XIII-2453r1-13
33. P. Sheehy et.al.: The black belt memory jogger: a pocket guide for six sigma success. ISBN-10 1576810437, ISBN 13-978-1576810439, Goal/QPC 1st edition, Jan 2002
34. E. Åstrand, Welding of heavy structures subjected to fatigue, Licentiate thesis, Cahlmers/Sweden 2013, ISBN 1652-8891
35. I. Lotsberg, Assessment of the size effect in fatigue analysis of butt welds and cruciform joints, Proceedings of the ASME 2014 33rd International Conference on Ocean, Offshore and Arctic Engineering OMAE2014 June 8-13, 2014, San Francisco, USA

Chapter 6
Root Side Requirements

6.1 General

When designing a weld, it is often desirable that the root side has a greater or at least the same fatigue life as the toe side. The reason is that weld toe cracking is visually easier to detect compared to root cracking. Also, a repair is generally more difficult to perform on a root crack compared to a toe crack. For more information on weld root design, see Ref. [1].

6.2 Joints with Weld Root as Weakest Point

Following the principles of "design for purpose," the analysis should focus on the identification of the weak points of the weld (toe or root) when loading is applied to the component, see also Chap. 2.4. In such an approach, there is a big difference between load-carrying and non-load-carrying welds. A butt weld should always be regarded being load-carrying since the loads and stresses pass through the weld. For fillet welds, the variations are bigger and some may be regarded as non-load-carrying while others must be regarded as fully load-carrying, which thus have the highest requirements. Whichever case, one could state that for load-carrying cases, the root side commonly becomes critical, while for non-load-carrying cases, the toe side often is critical. It is thus important to focus on parameters governing the stress levels in these points.

6.3 Designation for Penetration

When a weld is designed and given the designations on the drawing, it is common to state the quality level according to some standard, mostly ISO 5817. Further, for a fillet joint, the throat size needs to be stated. And in many cases, this is all stated and if so this implies a weld root-side designation which may become unclear.

B. Jonsson et al., *IIW Guidelines on Weld Quality in Relationship to Fatigue Strength*, IIW Collection, DOI 10.1007/978-3-319-19198-0_6

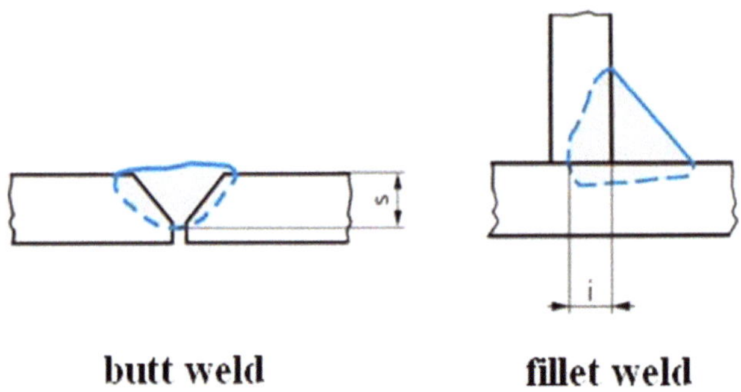

Fig. 6.1 Definition of weld partial penetration, "*s*" for butt joints and "*i*" for fillet joints

In order to reach a more detailed designation, it is important that the weld back side is addressed and this can be made through specification of the penetration, see Fig. 6.1.

If the partial penetration is considered in design process of welded joints, then the value of the penetration should be described as a requirement on the drawing, either as an *s*-measure for a butt weld or as an *i*-measure for a fillet weld. It can be given along with all other designations so that it is clear in the work shop which of the demands to focus on during welding.

In this way, it becomes possible for the designers to differentiate the requirements on the different parts of the weld: If the weld root side is critical, then attention can be given to the needed penetration and if the weld outside (toe) is critical, then attention can be given to the quality level. Following the principle of "design and weld for purpose," this can lead to a weld designation on the drawing, which is varied along the weld. This may be used to reach a longer fatigue life in high-stressed parts and lower welding cost in low-stressed areas.

To understand the influence of different parameters on the weld fatigue life, it is of interest to get an overview of how they act. Below, an attempt to show this is given as a variation of parameters and their influence on the weld root side. The analysis is made using the effective notch method [5] and the results are presented according to the theory for design of experiments (DoE), see Ref. [2].

6.4 Design of Experiments on an Example of Load-Carrying Weld

Consider a load-carrying cruciform joint and a welded butt joint, both cases having load-carrying characteristics. These cases will probably show a critical point at the root side if tension is applied. The weld toe might also be critical depending on the weld parameters and quality levels but this is not shown here.

These situations can be studied by applying the methods in design of experiments (DoE) and make use of simulations. DoE methods are typically and in general used for physical test setups, where many parameters have an effect on the result and where a full test setup varying all parameters is too expensive or time-consuming. In such a case, using DoE theories, it is possible to reduce the number of tests and still get valuable information of the important parameters. But this method can also be utilized by replacing the physical tests with simulations. In such a case a full test setup can be used since all needed is a parametric model and computer time. The simplest way is to vary the interesting parameters at two (2) levels, one high and one low, preferably with values on each side of the common or nominal one.

By combining all N parameters and vary them one at a time (resulting in 2^N computer simulations) the results can be studied statistically finding out what their individual influence is on the result. One can also see any combined effect between them, if there is one. Adding all results (notch stresses in this case), including signs (minus for “low” and plus for “high” level) and then averaging, gives the so-called effect and reveals the influence from a certain parameter. If a positive summary is reached, then an increase in this parameter increases the stress in the joint and if a negative summary is reached, then an increase in this parameter decreases the stress in the joint. Consequently, if the sum for a certain parameter is near zero or “small,” then this parameter has a low importance and vice versa. The parameters (or combinations of parameters) with a “small” effect in the stress level will be regarded as scatter (and could be compared to the scatter one get in physical tests). This is done by calculating the standard deviation (Stdv) of all effects, so a parameter may be regarded as significant if an effect is greater than say one (1) Stdv.

The described DoE method above has been carried out for two butt welds and a load-carrying cruciform joint and the result is shown in Figs. 6.2, 6.3, and 6.4, respectively.

The result indicates that for the butt joints, the only main effect is the lack of penetration (s-measure), if not full penetration is at hand. The thickness has some effect, even though not so high: The stress level will decrease when the thickness is increased.

For the load-carrying fillet weld, the penetration and the throat size are significant and both should be increased since the effect is negative (implying a stress decrease effect). The thickness is also significant, but has a positive effect, which means that the stress level increases when the thickness is increased and this is probably due to the fact that the root defect size increases (root defect = $t - 2i$). The effect is the opposite compared to the butt joint above. Misalignment, angle, undercut, and toe radius play a very small role for obvious reasons.

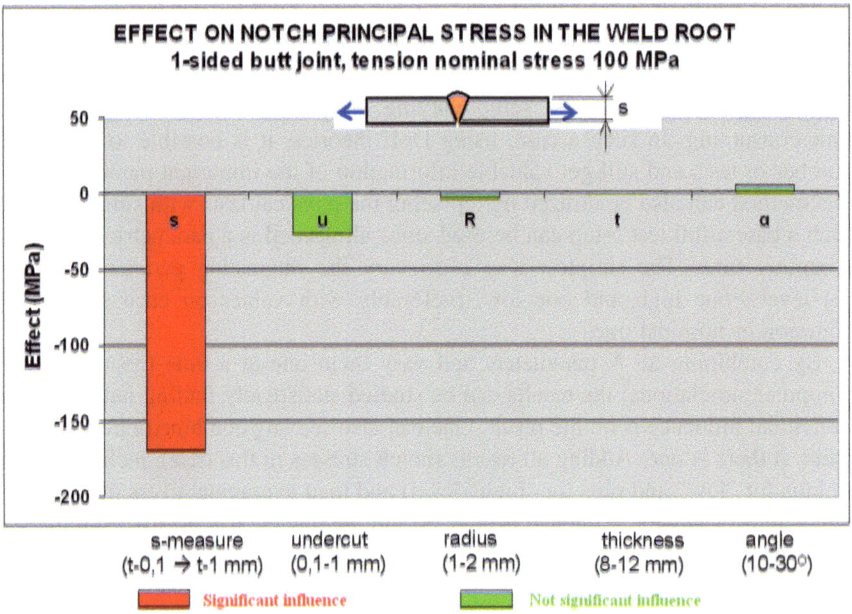

Fig. 6.2 Computed effects in weld root of a 1-side-welded butt joint

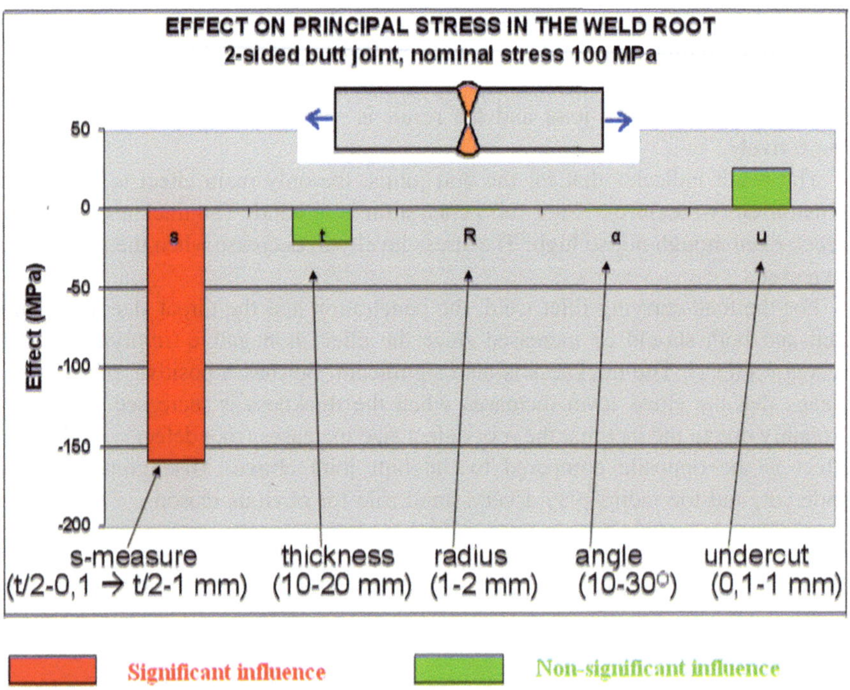

Fig. 6.3 Computed effects in weld root of a 2-side-welded butt joint

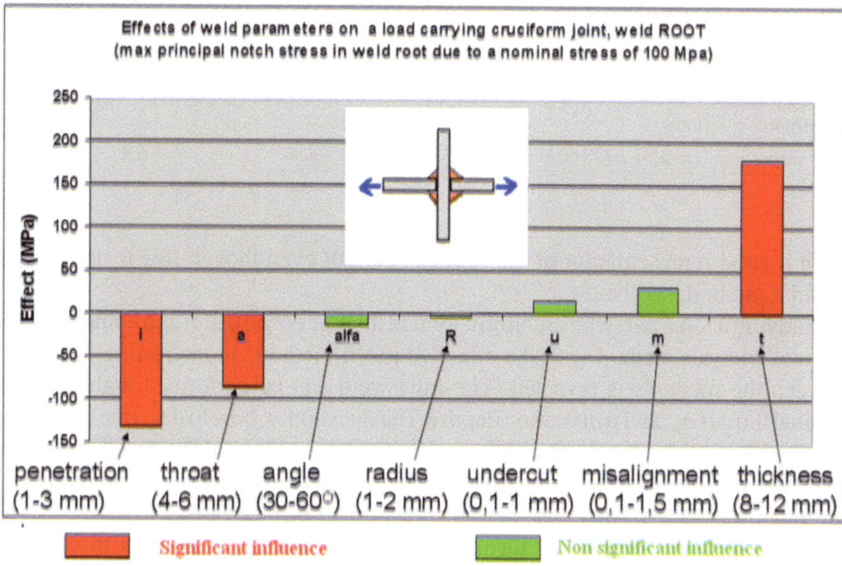

Fig. 6.4 Computed effects in weld root of a load-carrying cruciform joint

6.5 Throat Size Versus Penetration

As shown above for fillet joints, the penetration is the most important parameter for weld root fatigue followed by the throat size and of course the thickness itself, see Figs. 6.4 and 6.5. However, the parameters cannot be translated into each other directly, for instance, an increase of 1 mm penetration in a fillet weld is often worth much more than 1 mm more throat size (see Ref. [3] where 1 mm more penetration approximately equals 2 mm less nominal throat size regarding fatigue life). Many times the max (or sometimes called total) throat size a_{tot}, which includes both nominal throat a_n, and the penetration i, is used as a combined effect. However, this

Fig. 6.5 Fillet weld with partial penetration

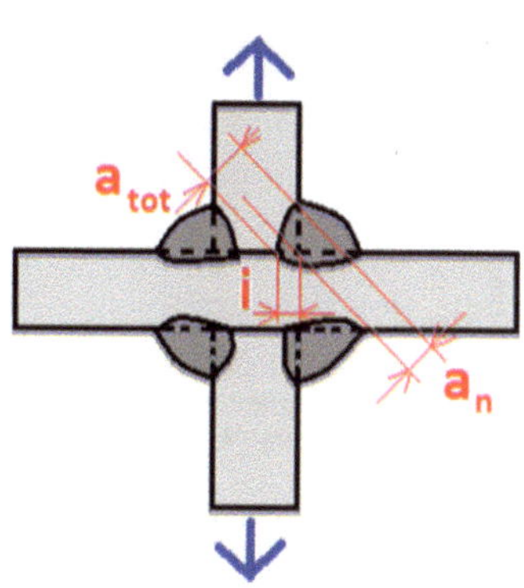

Table 6.1 Three different weld throat sizes (WTS) for t = 10 mm

	Optimized WTS	Ordinary WTS	Excessive WTS
Nominal throat = a_n (mm)	4	5	6.4
Penetration = i (mm)	3.4	2	0
Max throat = $a_{tot} = a_n + i/\sqrt{2}$ (mm)	6.4	6.4	6.4

is not a good representation of the fatigue strength even though this is used in the nominal method, see below.

Studying a *load-carrying* cruciform joint in thickness t = 10 mm and comparing the nominal analysis method with the effective notch method, an interesting difference between the methods is revealed. The fillet weld can be performed with different nominal throats $\boldsymbol{a_n}$, and penetration depth $\boldsymbol{i}$. The question is, how to describe this on the drawing? Usually a throat size only is given and nothing is expressed about the penetration. However, there is a need to do that and this can be shown in an example by studying three cases, which has the same max throat $\boldsymbol{a_{tot}}$ (see Table 6.1).

The analysis of these cases for the nominal method using the max throat, $\boldsymbol{a_{tot}}$, gives no difference, neither for the weld toe (FAT 71 without misalignment) nor for the weld root (FAT 36) (see Ref. [4]). The latter point depends on the fact that the nominal method uses the max throat, which is the same in all three cases. However, using the notch method, [5], there will be a difference (for both root and toe) since a load-carrying weld with higher penetration will have a better stress path through the weld. Assuming that the notch method results are correct (stress range 225 equivalent to 2E6 cycles), the stresses can be "back"-computed into the nominal world to see what would have been the applied nominal stress for the same fatigue life (2E6 cycles) (see colored columns in Fig. 6.6). The IIW Recommendation

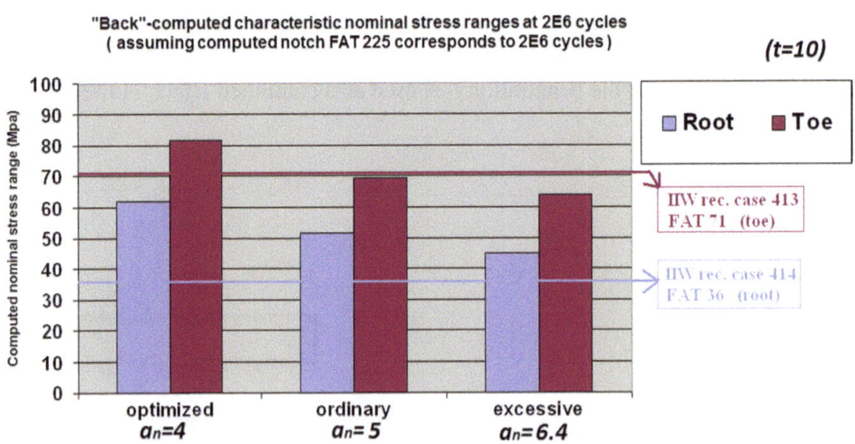

Fig. 6.6 "Back"-computed nominal stress ranges at 2E6 cycles for cruciform joint with 3 different nominal throat thicknesses (but same max or total throat)

nominal FAT levels are also given for toe and root, respectively, as lines for comparison. Note that the notch stress method includes a "thinnes" effect while this is not done in the nominal method for $t < 25$ mm and this explains some of the differences.

Looking at the results, one can firstly see that the joint in general has the lowest strength on the root side. The nominal FAT 36 is well below the computed levels in all three cases, implying a conservative design using this method. However, using the notch method, one can utilize quite a big improvement taking the penetration into account: For the optimized joint, a computed stress range of 62 MPa could be compared to FAT 36, implying a life increase of approximately 5 times: $(62/36)^3 \approx 5.1$.

On the weld toe side, the ordinary joint agrees well with the nominal FAT 71; however, for the excessive one, a non-conservative result could be the case using the nominal method if not FAT 63 would be assumed (note that the computation model has no misalignment included).

Another interesting observation is that the optimized weld joint, having the smallest nominal throat size and probably the best productivity in the work shop (lowest welding time and lowest amount of consumables), also has the highest fatigue performance on both weld toe and weld root side. This is one reason to include a penetration in the weld designations on the drawing and take this into account during the design of the joint using the effective notch method.

References

1. W. Fricke, Recommendation for the Fatigue Assessment of Weld Root Fatigue, IIW - XIII-2380r3-11/1383r3-11
2. P. Sheehy et.al.: The black belt memory jogger: a pocket guide for six sigma success. ISBN-10 1576810437, ISBN 13-978-1576810439, Goal/QPC 1st edition, January 2002.
3. K.E. Olsson, et.al. High strength welded box beams subjected to torsion and bending fatigue loads, Proceeding of conference *Welded High-Strength Steel Structures,* Stockholm Oct 1997, p.179-197.
4. A. Hobbacher, Recommendations for fatigue design of welded joints and components, IIW Document XIII-2151r1-07
5. W. Fricke Guideline for the Fatigue Assessment by Notch Stress Analysis for Welded Structures, IIW-Doc. XIII-2240r1-08/XV-1289r1-08

Chapter 7
Inspection, Quality Control, and Documentation

Fatigue in welds is to a great extent governed by geometric issues. This includes not only the local size of things in the weld but also all kinds of irregularities and imperfections that can be found and which are named in the language of the workshop as defects. The systems of weld quality levels, see for instance reference 4 in Chap. 4 [ISO 5817], describes imperfections normally found in welds. This means that weld quality systems are the most suitable tool to describe quality levels with reference to fatigue. Inspections made in a workshop also normally use these systems to determine whether the produced component fulfills the requirement stated on the drawing.

There are many situations where inspection is made, but one distinction can be made according to when it is performed compared to production. In short, the situations can be divided into different categories (see Table 7.1).

Quality assurance as part of the design phase of a weld is made during the prototype stage, when design and production together are working on new product and weld designs not earlier tried or where less experience exists or when the welding processes are changed to a great extent. Small samples are manufactured and studied preferably by cutting and sectioning to see whether they fulfill targets, i.e., fitness for use.

When production at a later stage is at full speed, the weld engineers and people on the workshop floor need to study the produced components in order to see that the weld looks all right. This situation could be named quality *control* and is more the type of a light inspection on more or less all components produced and the quality level which is asked for. It can be performed also based on a batch control as long as the quality is statistically assured. The visual inspection can be supported—depending on the quality level asked for—by NDT technology. It is to separate between detection and sizing of surface-breaking and inner imperfections. In the case of detection and sizing of surface-breaking imperfections, NDT technology is available on the basis of magnetic flux leakage (MT, magnetic particle inspection

B. Jonsson et al., *IIW Guidelines on Weld Quality in Relationship to Fatigue Strength*, IIW Collection, DOI 10.1007/978-3-319-19198-0_7

Table 7.1 Inspection schemes during the life of a welded product. Inspection techniques: VT visual, MT magnetic particle, PT penetrant testing, ET eddy current, RT radiographic, UT ultrasonic

Inspection category	When	Where	How
Quality assurance as a part of the design phase or optimization cycle	Prototype or optimization stage	New product development or during introduction of new welding processes	Destructive testing including sectioning, micrographs, and metallographic inspection
Quality control during production	During serialproduction	All welds in general	Visual inspection (VT) by the welding personnel and the supervisor. Depending on the quality level, the visual inspection is supported by NDT for detection and sizing of surface-breaking (MT, PT, ET) and inner imperfections in the volume (RT, UT)
Quality control after production or in-service	After a predetermined time period perhaps in the shop or on-site	May be all welds or selected welds depending on the component	Visual inspection (VT) by the welding and/or inspection personnel. Depending on the quality level, the visual inspection is supported by NDT for detection and sizing of surface-breaking (MT, PT, ET) and inner imperfections in the volume (RT, UT)
Revision to verify a process	After serialproduction has begun	Welds critical on drawing	Same tools as above

when the material is ferromagnetic), on the basis of penetration of colored or fluoroscopic liquids (PT), or on the basis of scanning with eddy current probes (ET). ET as inspection technology is mainly applied at non-magnetic welds and joints, for instance, in aerospace industry at laser-welded Al alloy structures as well as at riveted lap joints.

Depending on the safety level of a welded structure, laws in certain countries, codes, standards, and guidelines ask for an in-service inspection by NDT in predetermined time intervals, also defining the depth of inspection (for instance 50 % of all welds in 4 years). In that case, the same—above-mentioned techniques—are to apply, but depending on the safety level (for instance in aerospace, nuclear, and other pressure vessels using industries), high-sophisticated NDT technology can be asked for. However, all these techniques of which in many cases no standards not yet exist have to be qualified by qualification bodies asking for so-called performance demonstrations according to given consensus guidelines of the applying industry.

In mass production of serial goods, inspection must be made from time to time, called *revision* (or audition). This revision is part of a feedback process control

Table 7.2 Available standardized testing techniques

Location in the weld	Nondestructive testing (NDT)	Destructive testing (DT)
Outside	VT, MT, PT, replica, ET	Cutting, metallography, fatigue tests, fracture of samples
Inside of the weld (non-visible)	UT, RT	Cutting, metallography, fatigue tests, fracture of samples
Root side	UT, RT	Cutting, metallography, fatigue tests, fracture of samples

strategy to check process stability and quality of the optimized processes. Normally, this revision is not made on all produced components. Instead, some components are chosen randomly and studied by trained people, and these are comparing the real welds with the designations and specifications on the drawing in order to see whether the weld quality is fulfilled. The system used in this inspection is the so-called weld quality levels or weld class system, which have stated levels of different imperfections equivalent to different quality levels (see ISO 5817). The standardized techniques available are listed in Table 7.2.

7.1 Probability of Detection (POD) and Probability of Sizing (POS)

The modern methodology of NDT characterizes the ability to detect a specific imperfection of a given size (according to defect classes), which typically can occur in randomly fluctuating production processes by the well-defined term POD (probability of detection).

Figure 7.1 shows an example of POD curves, where schematically the POD in case of different NDT techniques [MP refers to magnetic particle inspection (MT), and US I-III refers to 3 different ultrasonic techniques (UT)] is discussed as a function of a geometry parameter of the imperfection, for instance, a crack size.

The methodology on which the determination of POD curves as shown in Fig. 7.1 is based is the comparison of a detected NDT indication, called â, with the real defect size, called a, revealed and confirmed by destructive tests. This needs the performance of a statistical investigation, taking into account a number of some thousand destructive sectioning tests with micrographs. The statistically determined correlation of â versus a has to be confirmed. However, Fig. 7.1 documents the POD in terms of real defect size a, confirmed by the destructive tests. This can only be the crack length in the case of NDT techniques such as MT or PT, which cannot indicate any crack depth. By the use of ET and UT techniques—depending on the

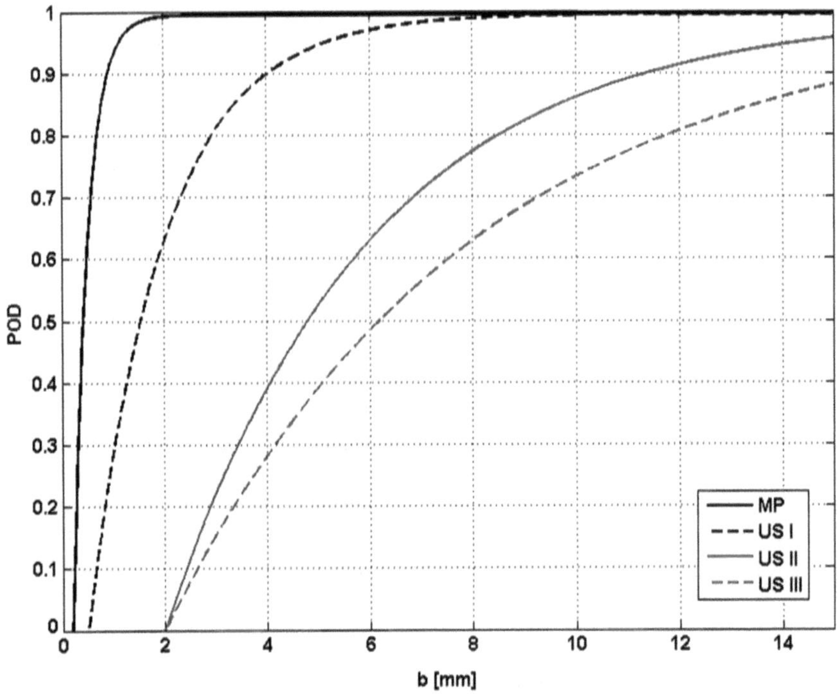

Fig. 7.1 POD as function of imperfection size, here, for example, crack size b in mm [MP refers to magnetic particle test (MT), US I-III refers to 3 different ultrasonic tests (UT)]

selected inspection parameters—crack depth profiles, as well as indication length and/or 3D indication images, can be evaluated as long as the NDT technique has imaging ability.

One important value characterizing the reliability of the NDT technique is the so-called $a^{90/95}$ value of imperfection size which indicates exactly the defect size which is detected with a probability of 90 % and this within a confidence interval of 95 %. The value, in aerospace industry, is the individual limit of detectability. The detectability asked for by the authorities for the detection of specified defects and the applied NDT technology has to be higher than this value.

These values are indicated in the Figs. 7.2 and 7.3, which document, in case of two different inspection teams, the performance obtained by POD calculation of the statistical data after phased array inspection. Both teams have measured the same set of specimen with hidden (unknown imperfections) at austenitic stainless steel welds. Team I has the lower $a^{90/95}$ value (8.046 mm)—i.e., a better detectability compared with Team II (8.926 mm)—but the scatter in the data is higher.

The POD can be enhanced by the optimization of the inspection technology [2]. Such an enhancement can be performed for instance in UT on carbon steel material

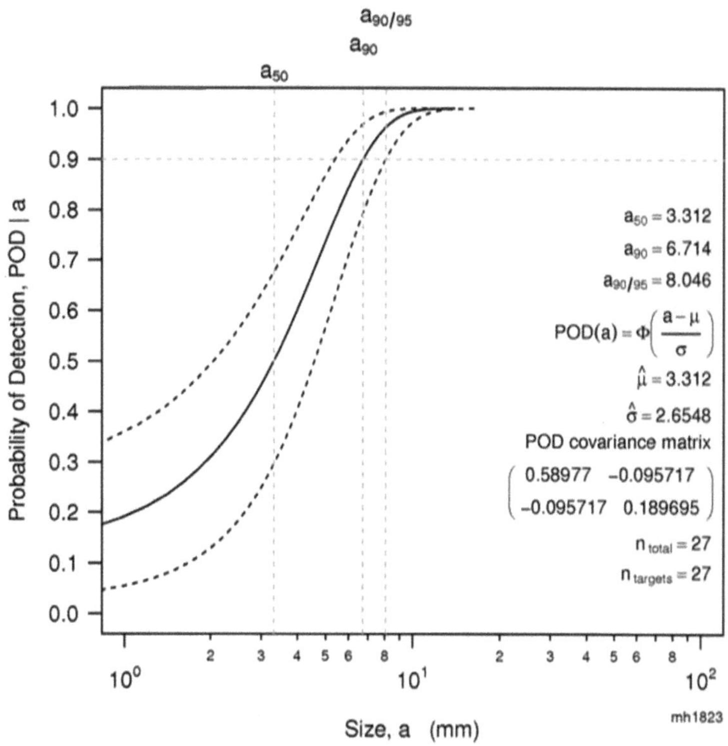

Fig. 7.2 UT by a phased array transducer at austenitic welds; Inspection Team I; the size a is the defect detection length [1]

by using a higher frequency, respectively, a shorter wave length or a focused transducer or signal enhancement and signal evaluation techniques, for instance, called synthetic aperture focusing technique (SAFT [3]), time-of-flight diffraction (TOFD [3]), full or half matrix capture-phased array in combination with SAFT and total focusing [4–6]. In any case, the signal enhancing strategy (online or in a post-processing analysis) is to reduce noise (electrical but also material structural noise), i.e., to enhance the signal-to-noise ratio and the spatial resolution. Noise is not only produced by the electronic noise of the equipment or structural noise (grain scattering, high attenuation) but by other influence parameters too. So it is well known [7] that enhanced surface roughness reduces the detectability of MT and PT by reducing the contrast between the imperfection indication and the background indication. A reduction of the imperfection indication is also observed in MT when the thickness of a corrosion protective paint is too large, and therefore, the magnetic field leakage amplitude in case of larger liftoff is reduced.

It should be mentioned here that POD curves are determined experimentally by collecting a lot of statistical data. Therefore, the curves always are superimposed by a scatter band, and confidence intervals can only be statistically evaluated (Figs. 7.2

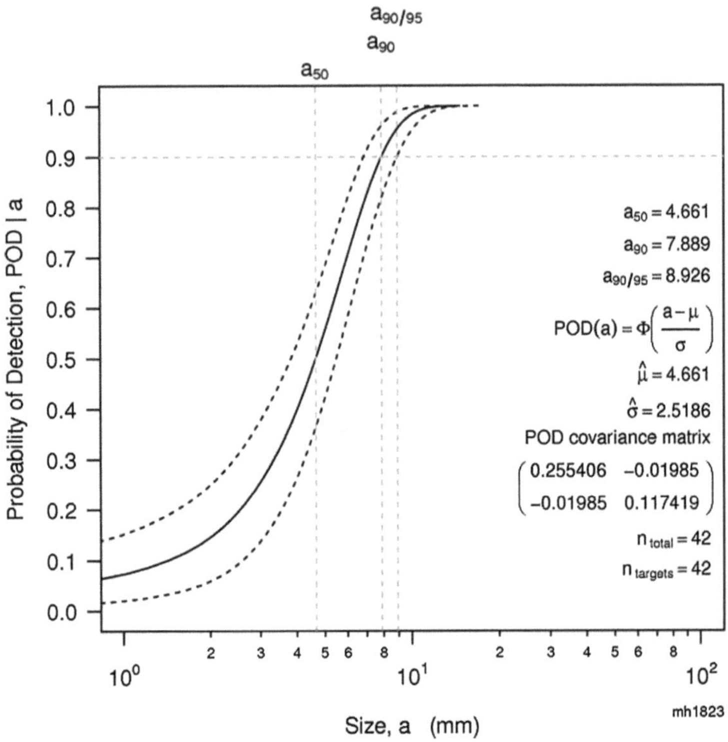

Fig. 7.3 UT by a phased array transducer at austenitic welds; Inspection Team II; the size a is the defect detection length [1]

and 7.3). Furthermore and mentioned above, the aerospace industry in maintenance generally asks for a detectability higher than characterized by the $a^{90/95}$ value. Therefore, the POD concepts were well documented in the field of aerospace [Ref MIL HDBK 1823]. Another fact is—see the tendency of PND in Fig. 7.4—the probability to "mishit" defects with large size is not zero and this is the critical case in safety-relevant NDT applications [1]. Safety has to be guaranteed not only by NDT application but generally by organizing an excellent quality management during the design phase, the construction phase, the commissioning phase, and in the service phase by lifetime management. In terms of the Bayesian terminology [8], one has to evaluate the "hit-rate" (true-positive calls and false-negative calls), the "mishit-rate" (true-negative calls), and the false alarm rate (false-positive calls). Whereas the true-negative calls (an imperfection exists but is not detected) are safety relevant and critical for live and environment, the false-positive calls (an imperfection is indicated but is not existing or is oversized) produce high costs by the initiation of really un-needed repair measures.

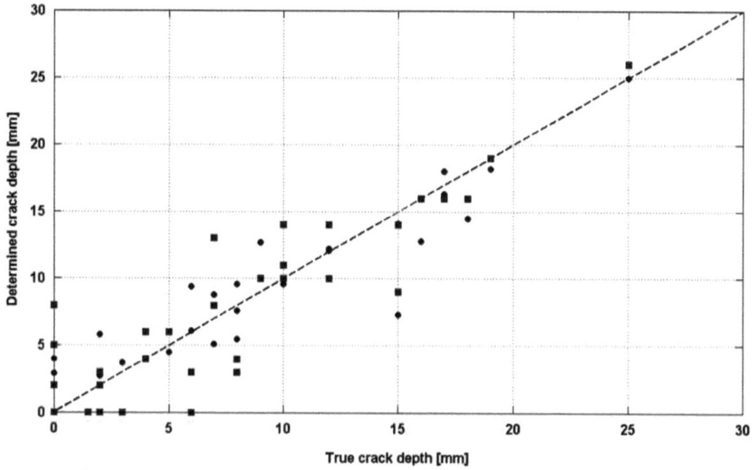

Fig. 7.4 Human factor influence of two inspection teams, scatter in the statistical data, imperfection size â determined by the teams versus the exact (true) size a [1]

7.2 Imperfection-Specific and NDT Technique-Specific POD

Concerning the specific NDT technique selected, different POD curves are found when different individual imperfections are inspected and each of them has to be discussed then also individually. As known from physical measurement processes, each measurement value is corrupted by measurement errors and an important task is to evaluate the error influences. Some of them are belonging to the measurement sensors and the measurement hardware and software; some come from the measurement procedure, i.e., its performance itself. What is true in case of measurement errors is valid for uncertainty of NDT too. Technology where only the costs of application are known but not its reliability will not be used. R&D in NDT actually is very much concentrated on the determination of POD and reliability in general.

7.3 Human Factor Influences

As long as human persons as inspectors are involved, a strong human factor influence has to be taken additionally into account. That is why in safety-relevant applications, for instance in the nuclear field, not only the technique (hardware and software) but also the inspection team is evaluated in blind tests in inspection qualification procedures [9] and a predetermined POD has to be achieved by the full team and its system of inspection. Figure 7.4 documents the fact in the case of the statistical data of the two teams of which the POD results were discussed in Figs. 7.2 and 7.3. The imperfection size determined by the teams is compared with the exact size obtained by reference investigation, for instance by metallography and sectioning of the component. Clearly, the human factor influence is revealed. However, both teams have also used different commercial phased array systems and this influence factor is also superimposed.

7.4 Real-Time Inspection

There exist some NDT techniques which allow an online or real-time inspection during the welding or joining procedure. Examples for such techniques are the monitoring of multilayer submerged arc welding by acoustic emission which many years ago [10] was introduced in the USA in nuclear industry or the active UT through transmission in case of electrical resistance spot welding [11]. An actual NDT technology under development is due to online monitoring of laser welding fillet welds in case of ship desks [12]. The UT transducer used is a so-called electromagnetic acoustic transducer (EMAT, [13, 14]). Its advantage is to have no need of an acoustic coupling media, and therefore, it can be applied even at elevated temperatures of the inspection product. Figure 7.5 shows a micrograph of a fillet weld indicating a LOF defect which was not detected by applying RT.

In Fig. 7.6, a so-called C-scan inspection image is shown. This image is obtained when the EMAT is moved parallel along the weld in a fixed distance by a mechanical manipulation and insonifying the weld by an ultrasound beam perpendicular to the weld. However, the NDT technology is not yet available and is under further development.

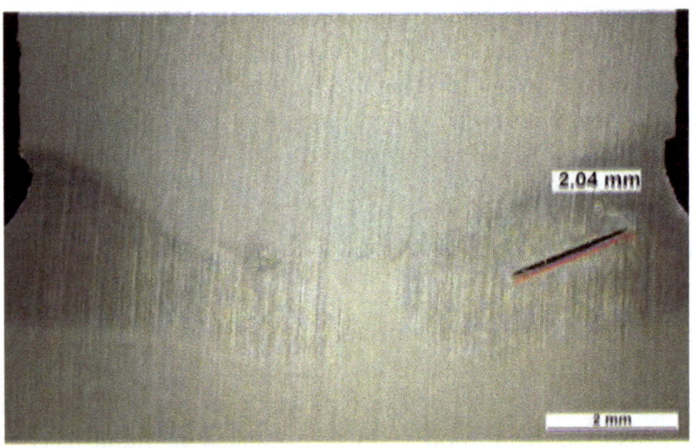

Fig. 7.5 A LOF (lack-of fusion) imperfection of 2.04-mm crack length, not detected by RT

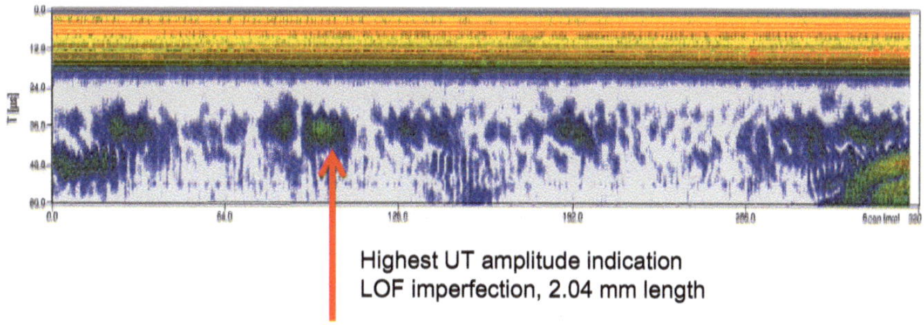

Fig. 7.6 UT indication by EMAT

7.5 Notes on Limits

This § was written in collaboration with sub commission VC chaired by Daniel CHAUVEAU—Institut de Soudure.

The described limits of detectability of the above-mentioned main NDT techniques and the most relevant imperfections (surface and inner imperfections such as root defect (partial penetration), undercuts, pores, toe radius, surface defects, cold laps, misalignments, and throat size) have limits. These limits of detectability are given in Table 7.3 in the following. However, it should be mentioned that these limits are given under the assumption of the best case concerning influencing parameters producing a reduced signal-to-noise ratio; i.e., signal-to-noise ratio has to be higher than 6 dB, and the average surface roughness value has to be lower than 8 μm.

Also, when inspection is being used, it is of importance that the technique is statistically secured. This can be investigated in a measurement system analysis (MSA), where the inspection is tested to see whether a result can be repeated (same person inspects same weld on different occasions) and reproduced (different persons inspects a weld). A method could be said to be approved if the so-called Kendall coefficient (ranging from 0 to 1) is above 0.90 (see Ref. [17]).

The physical flaw descriptions of EN ISO 5817 do not equate to the capabilities of different NDT techniques to detect, discriminate, and size certain types of imperfections.

CEN/TC 121 and TC 54 have agreed that there is a fundamental difference between quality level as defined in EN ISO 5817 and acceptance levels as defined in NDT EN ISO standard. NDT does not size the physical flaw, but the indication results in the interaction of a physical principle with the flaw. EN ISO 17635 specifies how to rely quality level to acceptance levels. The main ISO weld standards to apply are summarized in the following Table 7.4.

Inspection procedures are made up of a mix of NDT techniques, setting procedures or calibrating principles, decision steps, scanning systems, recording, and illustration tools and software. They often involve a process of interpretation of

Table 7.3 State of the art for the detection of different imperfections

Name and N° ISO 6520-1	Sketch	VT and gauges	l	h	RT	l	h	UT	l	h	First technique to apply
External Undercut (butt weld) (5011)	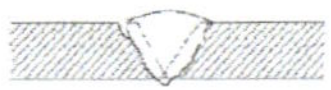	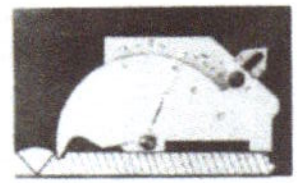	1	1	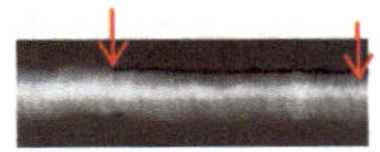	1	0	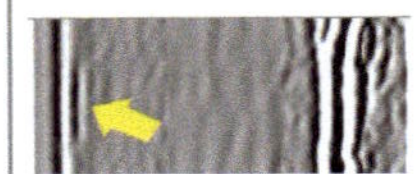	1	3	VT
Internal Undercut (butt weld) (5013)	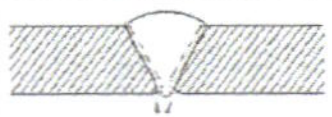	Possible by means of a borescope (backside access required)	2	2 (a)	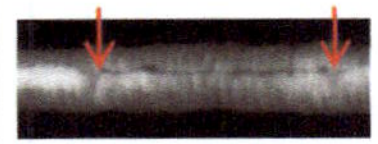	1	0	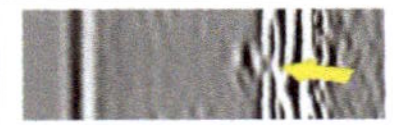	1	3	VTUT (if no backside access)
Undercut (fillet weld) (5011)	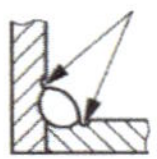	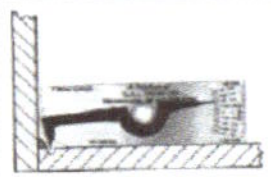	1	1		2	0		1	3	VT
Misalignment (507)	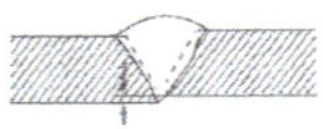	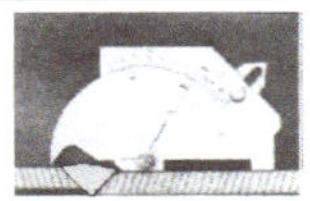 (after-welding)	1	1	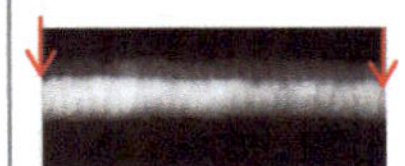	1	0		2	3	VTUT TOFD (if no backside access)
		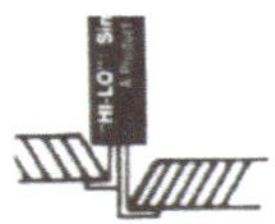 (before-welding)	1	1							
Reinforcement	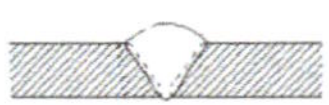	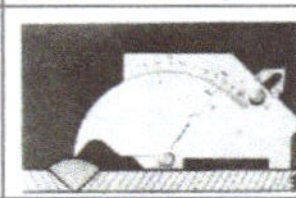	1	1	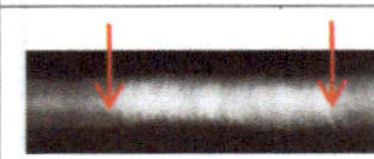	1	0		0	0	VT

(continued)

Table 7.3 (continued)

Name and N° ISO 6520-1	Sketch	VT and gauges	l	h	RT	l	h	UT	l	h	First technique to apply
Fillet leg length	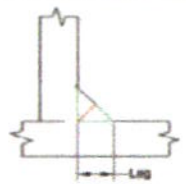	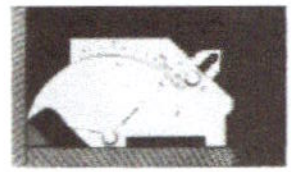	1	/		3	/		2	/	VT
Fillet weld throat	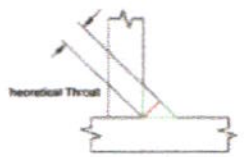	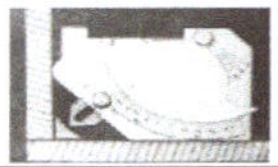	/	1		/	0		/	3	VT
Incomplete penetration fillet weld	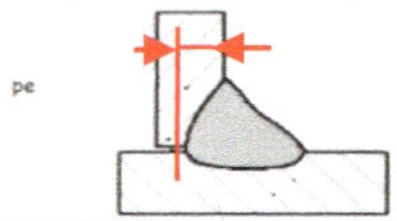		0	0		3	3		3	3	Tomography UT
Incomplete root penetration butt weld	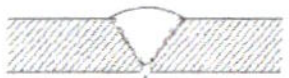	Possible by means of a borescope (backside access required)	2	2 (a)	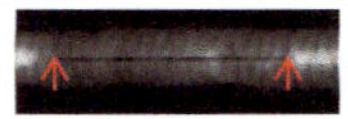	1	3		1	2 3	RT (UT if h is requested)
Embedded pores (2011)	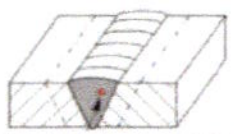	Not possible	0	0	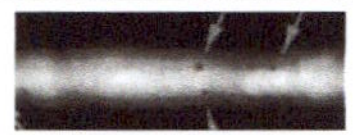	1	3		3	3	RT (tomography if h is requested)
Surface pores (2017-2018)	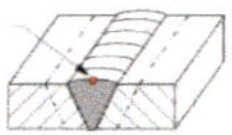	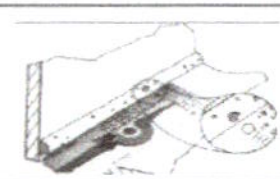	1 (c)	2	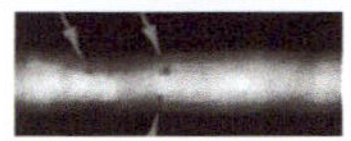	1	3		3	3	VT (tomography if h is requested)
Surface breaking cracks (101)	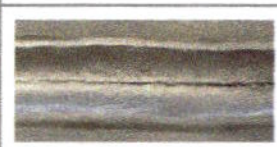		1 (c)	0	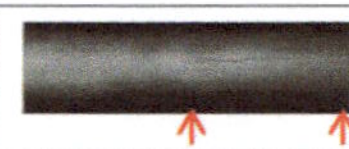	2	3	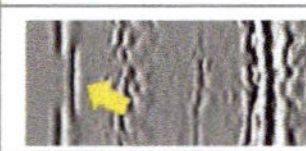	1	2 3	UT
Embedded crack (101)	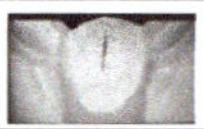		0	0	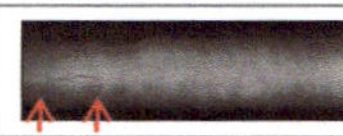	2	3	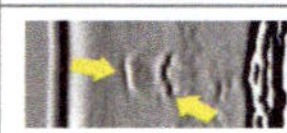	1	2 3	UT

(continued)

Table 7.3 (continued)

Name and N° ISO 6520-1	Sketch	VT and gauges	l	h	RT	l	h	UT	l	h	First technique to apply
Root crack (101)	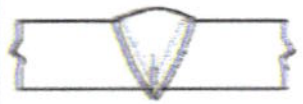	Possible by means of a borescope (backside access required)	2	0		2	3	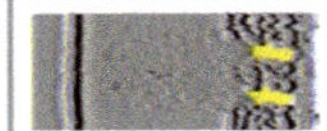	1	2 3	UT
Embedded cold crack	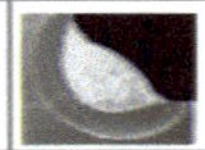		0	0		3	0		2 3	2 3	UT
Cold laps (506) (overlap)	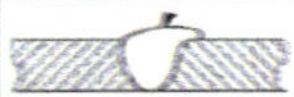	Detection possible by PT	0 (c)	0		0	0		0	0	PT

Name and N° ISO 6520-1	Sketch	VT and gauges	Angle	RT	Angle	UT	Angle	First technique to apply
Plate preparation angle		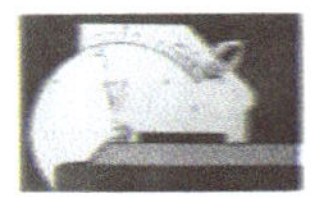	1		0		0	VT
Butt Weld surface angle (incorrect toe) (5051)	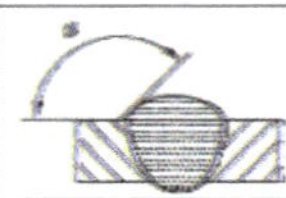	Gauge exists appropriate one should be selected	1		0		0	VT
Fillet Weld surface angle (incorrect toe) (5051)	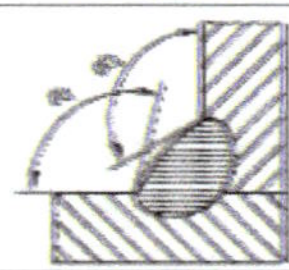	Gauge exists appropriate one should be selected	1		0		0	VT

(continued)

Table 7.3 (continued)

Name and N° ISO 6520-1	Sketch	VT and gauges	Angle	RT	Angle	UT	Angle	First technique to apply
Weld toe radius (5052)	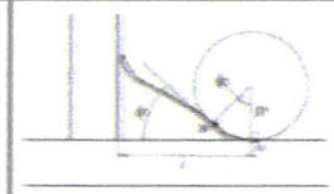	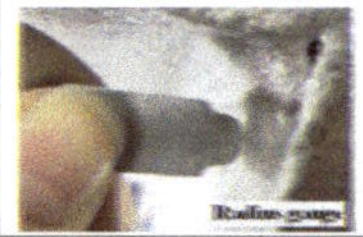	1 (b)		0		0	VT with gauges using pre-machined block + torch
Fillet weld geometries so far the weld surface is machined, for instance by grinding to an average roughness value Ra < 20 µm Actually no standards exist	**In comparison as an example**: Surface breaking cracks in a austenitic weave bead cladding and strip weld cladding on a ferritic base material [7.15]	**ET by an eddy current probe in combination with a manipulation for automatic scanning**	Detection limit (6 dB higher than noise) 3 mm deep, 10 mm long for weave bead cladding Detection limit (6 dB higher than noise) 2 mm deep, 20 mm long for strip weld cladding The noise signals here are due to lift-off fluctuations of the probe and due to δ-ferrite phases in the austenitic structure of the cladding The approach has its basis on the application of low frequencies in the 0.5–20 kHz-range.					

Legend
Colum l: gives the capability of the technique/method to assess the length of an indication or a leg of a fillet weld
Colum h: gives the capability of the technique/method to assess the height/depth of an indication (undercut …) or a geometrical weld feature extension (misalignment …)
/: not applicable
0: not possible
1: standard technique(s) may be used under all or most situation
2: standard technique(s) may be used under certain conditions
3: special technique(s), conditions and/or personnel qualification are required—doesn't work in all the condition/situation
Notes
(a) special device such a laser profiler shall be available on the boroscope equipment
(b) the use of a master block for calibration is required—Dental cement molding may be used
(c) surface method (PT—MT—ET should be applied)

Table 7.4 Standards for different nondestructive techniques

NDT method/technique	Abbreviation	Weld standard (methodology)	Weld standard (acceptance level)
Visual testing	VT	ISO 17637	ISO 5817
Radiographic testing (film)	RT	ISO 17636-1	ISO 10675-1&2
Ultrasonic testing (manual)	UT	ISO 17640	ISO 11666
Ultrasonic testing (TOFD)	TOFD(*)	ISO 10863	ISO 15626
Ultrasonic testing (phased array)	PA	ISO 13588	In progress
Penetrant testing	PT	ISO 3452-1	ISO 23777
Magnetoscopy testing	MT	ISO 17638	ISO 23278

Note (*) TOFD means time-of-flight diffraction technique

indications which relies on the skill of the operator. As a result [16], they cannot be considered simply as measurements and NDE performance for detecting, locating, and classifying and sizing defects cannot be represented by simple confidence intervals. Higher sophisticated POD procedures have to be taken into account.

VT: Visual technique is the oldest form of inspection. It may be performed by the naked eye or by aid of tools such as magnifying glasses, mirrors, and endoscopes. It is only used for the detection of surface defects. Inspection may be performed both from the outside and, with the aid of specialized tools such as endoscopes, from the inside of constructions. However, detection is limited to surface-breaking defects, and additional NDT is required when defects in the volume shall be detected. Visual inspection shows the shape and extent of surface anomalies. Since only the surface is viewed, only the surface indication dimensions can be measured generally by means of a ruler (accuracy ±1 mm); a large choice of welding gauges are available on the market. The choice shall be made in accordance with the objective of the inspection: checking alignment, checking dimensions before or after welding, verifying weld dimensions, and assessing surface-breaking defect. Some gauges are multipurpose or single purpose. Accuracy depends on gauge type and width of the surface-breaking defect.

Profilers (using laser or not) may be used instead of weld gauges. (Laser profilers are more expensive and generally not so versatile and can be limited on complex geometries such nozzles.) Their characteristics (resolution, accuracy, dimensions, etc.) shall be carefully chosen in accordance with the inspection objectives, available access, and software capabilities.

Surface NDT techniques such as magnetic testing (MT) or penetrant testing (PT) may be used to optimize detection and length assessment of surface defects.

ET: Eddy current testing is based on the fact that electric currents excited as eddy currents by an inductive coil are disturbed by crack-like and volumetric imperfections with other electrical conductivity than the host material. This can be detected by observing the coil impedance. The technique is widely introduced to inspect lap joints and riveted structures of air planes made of Al alloys. In the nuclear field, surface-breaking defects in austenitic steel (pipes and cladding) are detected. Concerning ferritic steels, a high disturbing noise is due to magnetic permeability changes. Here, only a multifrequency approach can be applied [15]. The application at fillet welds is not a standard inspection situation.

RT: Radiographic technique is one of the most commonly used methods for volumetric inspection. The energy of the source to be used depends on the thickness and type of material to be irradiated. An increasing wall thickness results in decreasing defect detectability. Also an appropriate choice of energy source and type of film greatly influences the detection of defects. The object may be irradiated with X-rays or gamma rays. The source is placed on one side of the object under inspection and the film on the other side. In this way, an image of the object is produced. A decrease of the irradiated thickness by the presence of a defect results in a higher density of radiation on the film directly underneath the defect. In this way, weld defects, cracks, casting cavities, and, to a certain extent, geometrical deviations may be detected. In principle, this technique is only suitable for detecting planar defects more or less aligned with the beam, when they can generate sufficient difference in the density of radiation on the film. RT can be used to detect defects in the volume of specimen as well as surface-breaking defects, in welds. It is well suited for the detection of voluminous defects such as cavities and porosity. RT is not capable of measuring the through-thickness height (h) of defects (special RT procedures using markers and/or several shots (i.e., parallax technique), and tomography can achieve this objective, but in that last case, the part to test shall be set in the tomographic chamber.

The length of a defect can be assessed with any significant accuracy only when it is well orientated and wide enough. RT is a very powerful tool because it enables when the imperfection is detected to give it a name.

UT: Ultrasonic techniques. Manual pulse echo ultrasonic technique (MUT), together with radiography, is among the most commonly used methods for volumetric inspection. It is more sensitive than radiography for the detection of planar defects, but the scope of inspection is limited (in standard) to parts having a thickness ≥8 mm. It is applicable to most construction materials, although some materials may be difficult to inspect due to coarse grain structure or anisotropic behavior, resulting in high "acoustical noise," damping, and beam deflection (e.g., austenitic steel, brass, and synthetic materials). Manual UT relies on the reflection of ultrasonic waves by imperfections in the material under testing, such as cavities, cracks, and weld defects. Pulse echo technique is a relative method; i.e., results are always related to signals obtained in a known situation (i.e., comparison is made with the signals received from reference reflectors such as holes and notches, a known wall thickness). Signal amplitude does not supply explicit information about the true height of a defect because the signal amplitude depends on more parameters than defect size alone, such as surface condition, defect type, and orientation relative to the ultrasonic incident beam. Defect length can be estimated with a reasonable degree of accuracy from the loss of signal as the probe is moved along the length of a defect. The wider the ultrasonic beam diameter, the greater the inaccuracy of the measurement of defect length.

When defect height shall be assessed, diffraction techniques shall be used (possible to be applied manually but the use of imaging UT techniques (TOFD, phased array, etc.) should be preferred). TOFD results appear in terms of indication position, length, and location in vertical direction. Defect height may be assessed when above a certain threshold, depending on the resolution with which signals from upper and lower tip can be separated (related to frequency and equipment resolution). Typical values for minimum height that can be resolved are 1–3 mm. Site accuracy for height measurement falls in the range of 1 mm.

References

1. http://www.sciencedirect.com/science/article/pii/S1350630713002082
2. G. Dobmann, D.D. Cioclov, J.H. Kurz; NDT and fracture mechanics. How we can improve failure assessment by NDT? Where we are – where we go. Insight Vol 53 No 12 December 2011, 668-672
3. M. Spies, Spies, Martin, H. Rieder, A. Dillhöfer, V. Schmitz; W. Müller: Synthetic Aperture Focusing and Time-of-Flight Diffraction ultrasonic imaging-past and present. J Nonderstruct Eval (2012), 31, 310-323
4. C. Holmes, B. Drinkwater, and P.D. Wilcox: Post-processing of the full matrix of ultrasonic transmit-receive array data for non-destructive evaluation. NDT & E International 38 (8) 2005, 701-711
5. A.J. Hunter, B.W. Drinkwater, and P.D. Wilcox: Autofocusing ultrasonic imagery for non-destructive testing and evaluation of specimens with complicated geometries. NDT & E International 43 (2), 2010, 78-85
6. J. Verkooijen, A. Bulavinov: Sampling phased array, a new technique for ultrasonic signal processing and imaging. Insight 50 (3) 2008, 153-157
7. Subcommission VE of Commission V of the IIW: Handbook on the magnetic examination of welds, Document IIS/IIW-849-87. The Welding Institute, Cambridge CB1 6AL, UK
8. D. Spiegelhalter, K. Rice: Bayesian Statistics, (2009), Scholarpedia, 4(8), 5230
9. P. Lemaitre et al.: The European methodology developed by ENIQ, Principles and implementation. 7th International Conference on Nuclear Engineering, ICONE-7011, Tokyo, Japan, April 19-23, 1999
10. P.H. Hutton, E.B. Schwenk, and R.J. Kurtz: Progress toweard acoustic emission characterization for continuous monitoring reactor pressure vessels. Proceedings of the International Symposium New Methods in NDE of Materials and their Application especially in Nuclear Engineering, Saarbrücken 17-19 September 1979, German Society for NDT (DGZfP), Berlin
11. K. Ofterdinger, E. Waschkies: Temperature-dependence of the ultrasonic transmission through electrical-resistance heated imperfect metal- metal interfaces. NDT&E International 37 (2004), Nr.5, 361-371
12. M. Dahmen, A. Drenker, Ch. Robert, W. Fiedler, M. Kirchhoff, T. Kring, M. Kogel-Hollacher, F. Niese, Ch. Paul, R. Wagener: Automation of Laser-Arc Hybrid Welding of 3D-Structures by Process Monitoring and Control. LANE 2012, www.elsevier.com/locate/procedia
13. H.J. Salzburger: EMATs and its Potential for Modern NDE - State of the Art and Latest Applications. Proceedings of the IEEE International Ultrasonics Symposium 1, 2009, 621-628
14. H.J. Salzburger, F. Niese, G. Dobmann: EMAT pipe inspection with guided waves. Welding in the world 56 (2012), 5-6, 35-43

15. R. Weiß, R. Becker. B. Lucht. F. Mohr, K. Hartwig: Qualification of the Low-Frequency (LF)-eddy current technique for the inspection of stainless steel cladding and applications on the reactor pressure vessel. Nuclear Engineering and Design 206 (2001), 311-223
16. The FITNET fitness-for-service thematic network – Annex D (NDE)
17. A. Ericson-Öberg: Improved quality assurance of fatigue loaded structures, Thesis for degree Licentiate, Chalmers University, Sweden, ISSN:1652-8891, April 2013

Chapter 8
Fitness for Service

Assessment of welds not meeting "standard" requirements may sometimes be of interest to investigate. An example is to determine the fatigue life from a found crack-like defect to failure. It is recommended to use local-based methods, such as the effective notch method or the fracture mechanics method with the guidance of well-established recommendations, e.g., BS 7910 or comparable ones.

8.1 General

Fracture mechanics is used for several purposes as follows:

(a) Assessment of fracture, especially brittle fracture, in a component containing cracks or crack-like details.
(b) Assessment of fatigue properties in a component containing cracks or crack-like imperfection, e.g., in welded joints.
(c) Predicting the fatigue properties of severely notched components with no or a relatively short crack initiation phase. Welded joints behave as being severely notched. Predictions are made assuming small initial defects.

The fatigue assessment procedure as in (b) and (c) is performed by the calculation of the growth of an initial crack a_i to a final size a_f. The parameter which describes the fatigue action at a crack tip in terms of crack propagation is the stress intensity factor (SIF) range ΔK. The starting crack configuration is the center crack in an infinite plate. The SIF K is defined by the formula $K = \sigma \cdot \sqrt{\pi \cdot a}$ where σ is the remote stress in the plate and a is the crack parameter, here the half distance from tip to tip.

In existing components, there are various crack configurations and geometrical shapes (see Fig. 8.1). So, corrections are needed for the deviation from the

B. Jonsson et al., *IIW Guidelines on Weld Quality in Relationship to Fatigue Strength*, IIW Collection, DOI 10.1007/978-3-319-19198-0_8

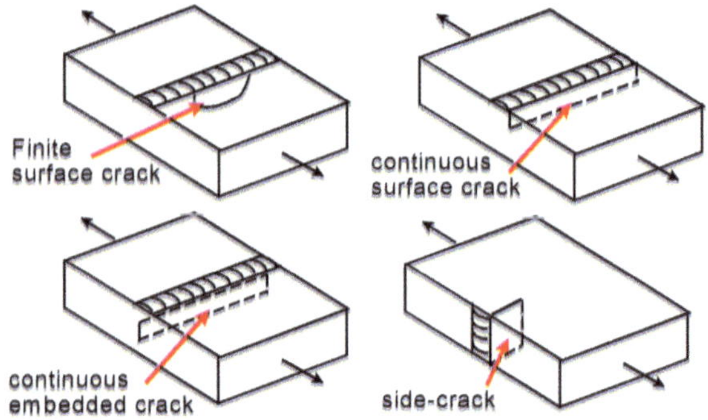

Fig. 8.1 Examples for different categories of cracks

center-cracked plate. These corrections take into account the following parameters and crack locations:

(a) Free surface of a surface crack,
(b) Embedded crack located inside of a plate,
(c) Limited width or wall thickness,
(d) Shape of a crack, mostly taken as being elliptic,
(e) Distance to an edge.

The formula for the SIF has due to this to be expanded by a correction function $Y_u(a)$ to

$$K = \sigma\sqrt{\pi \cdot a} \cdot (Y_u(a))$$

8.2 Stress Intensity Factors

8.2.1 General Solution

For a variety of crack configurations, parametric formulae for the correction function $Y_u(a)$ have been developed. These correction functions are based on different applied stress types (e.g., membrane, bending, structural hot spot stress, and nominal stress). The one used must correspond to the stress type under consideration.

8.2.2 Stress Intensity Factor for Welds

Fracture mechanics calculations related to welded joints are generally based on the total stress at the notch root, e.g., at the weld toe. The universal correction function $Y_u(a)$ may be separated into the correction of a standard configuration $Y(a)$ and an additional correction for the local notch of the weld toe $M_k(a)$. A further separation into membrane stress and shell bending stress was done at most of the parametric formulae for the functions $Y(a)$ and $M_k(a)$ [8–12].

In practical application, first the relevant applied stress (usually the local nominal or the structural hot spot stress) at the location of the crack is determined, assuming that no crack is present. In general, the stress should be separated into membrane and shell bending stress components. The SIF K then results as a superposition of the effects of both stress components. The effects of the crack shape and size are covered by the correction function Y. The effects of any remaining stress raising discontinuity or notch (nonlinear peak stress) can be covered by additional factors M_k, while

$$K = \sqrt{\pi \cdot a} \cdot \left(\sigma_m \cdot Y_m(a) \cdot M_{k,m}(a) + \sigma_b \cdot Y_b(a) \cdot M_{k,b}(a)\right)$$

where

K Stress intensity factor
σ_m Membrane stress
σ_b Shell bending stress
Y_m Correction function for membrane stress intensity factor
Y_b Correction function for shell bending stress intensity factor
$M_{k,m}$ Correction for nonlinear stress peak at the weld toe in terms of membrane action
$M_{k,b}$ Correction for nonlinear stress peak at the weld toe in terms of shell bending.

The correction functions Y_m and Y_b can be found in the literature. The solutions in refs. [1–6] are particularly recommended. For most cases, the formulae for SIFs given are adequate. M_k-factors may be found in Refs. [7, 8].

8.2.3 Weight Function Approach

The weight function approach is based on the idea that a given stress distribution can be discretized into differential pairs of split forces which open a crack. The action of each differential force on a crack can be described by a function, the so-called weight function $h(x,a)$. The determination of the SIF is thus reduced into an integration over the crack length. By this method, arbitrary stress distributions can be assessed [15, 16]. The basic formulation of the weight function approach is

$$K = \int_{x=0}^{x=a} \sigma(x) \cdot h(a,x) \cdot \mathrm{d}x$$

The weight function of a center crack in a plate is

$$h = \frac{2}{\sqrt{\pi}} \cdot \sqrt{\frac{a}{a^2 - x^2}}$$

and with the stress concentration factor $k_t(x) = \sigma(x)/\sigma_{\text{ref}}$ follows that

$$K = \frac{2}{\pi} \int_{x=0}^{x=a} \sigma(x) \cdot \sqrt{\frac{a}{a^2 - x^2}} \cdot \mathrm{d}x = \sigma_{\text{ref}} \cdot \sqrt{\pi \cdot a} \cdot \frac{2}{\pi} \int_{x=0}^{x=a} \frac{k_t(x)}{\sqrt{a^2 - x^2}} \cdot \mathrm{d}x$$

This solution for center crack in infinite plate and for an arbitrary stress distribution may also be used for the standard solutions (see chapters below). In that case, the correction formulae $Y(a)$ have to be applied.

$$K = \sigma_{\text{ref}} \cdot \sqrt{\pi \cdot a} \cdot Y(a) \cdot \frac{2}{\pi} \int_{x=0}^{x=a} \frac{k_t(x)}{\sqrt{a^2 - x^2}} \cdot \mathrm{d}x$$

This formula is sufficiently accurate at short cracks, and at longer cracks, accuracy will decrease. Since most of the fatigue life is spent at small cracks, this formula can be reasonably applied. It is also useful in determination of M_k functions, where $k_t(x)$ is the stress concentration factor distribution.

$$M_k = \frac{2}{\pi} \int_{x=0}^{x=a} \frac{k_t(x)}{\sqrt{a^2 - x^2}} \cdot \mathrm{d}x$$

More general and accurate weight functions have been developed for 2-dimensional [15] and 3-dimensional problems. Even more weight functions may be found in literature.

The application of weight functions requires an integration process to obtain the SIF. Here, it must be observed that several weight functions lead to improper integrals, i.e., integrals with infinite boundaries but finite solutions. There are two ways to overcome. Firstly to use very fine steps near the singularity, or secondly to integrate analytically, if possible, and to calculate small stripes, which are added later.

For transverse loaded welds, parametric formulae for the stress distribution in the plate have been developed. In these cases, a finite element calculation to derive the stress distribution is not necessary [19].

8.2.4 Finite Element Programs

Finite element programs may be used for the determination of stresses and stress distributions. It must be made sure that the refinement of the meshing corresponds to the method, which is used for deriving the SIFs.

For the use of standard solutions and existing M_k-formulae, a coarse meshing may be sufficient to determine the membrane and the shell bending stress. If a weight function approach is used, a finer meshing is needed for a complete information about the stress distribution at the weld toe.

Several program systems exist which provide a direct determination of SIFs. The meshing should be made according to the method used and to the recommendations of the program manual.

8.2.5 Aspect Ratio

The aspect ratio $a/2c$ is a significant parameter for the SIF, see Fig. 8.2. It has to be taken into consideration at fracture mechanics calculations. This consideration can be done in different ways:

(a) Direct determination and calculation of crack growth in c-direction, e.g., by 3-dimensional weight functions or M_k-formulae. These formulae give the SIFs at the surface, which governs the crack propagation in c-direction.
(b) Application of formulae and values which have been derived by fitting of experimental data, e.g., by Engesvik [13].

$$\begin{aligned} 2c &= -0.27 + 6.34a \quad && \text{if } a < 3\,\text{mm} \\ a/(2c) &= 0 && \text{if } a > 3\,\text{mm} \end{aligned}$$

(c) If only 2-dimensional Mk-values are given, then the crack depth of $a = 0.15$ mm (initiation) may be used as a conservative approach to calculate the effective SIF at the surface.
(e) A constant aspect ratio of $a{:}2c = 0.1$ may be taken as a conservative approach.

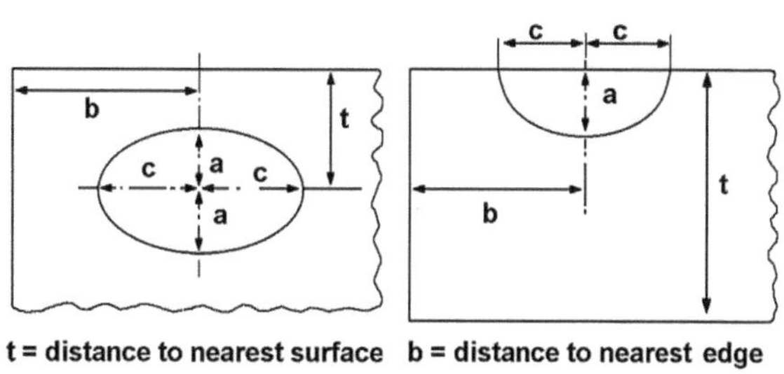

Fig. 8.2 Aspect ratio of cracks

8.2.6 Assessment of Welded Joints Without Detected Imperfections

Fracture mechanics may be used to assess the fatigue properties of welded joints in which no imperfections have been detected. In such cases, it is necessary to assume the presence of a crack, for example, based on prior metallurgical evidence or the detection limit of the used inspection method, and then to calculate the SIFs as described above.

For cracks starting from a weld toe, in absences of other evidence, it is recommended that an initial crack depth of $a = 0.05 \ldots 0.15$ mm and an aspect ratio as given above should be taken. These initial cracks have been derived from fitting the assessment procedure to existing experimental data, disregarding possible fracture mechanics short crack effects. If possible, the calculations should be compared or calibrated at similar joint details with known fatigue properties.

If no weld toe radius ρ was specified or determined by measuring, it is recommended to assume a sharp corner, i.e., a toe radius of $\rho = 0$ or $\rho = 0.2$ mm. For root gaps in load-carrying fillet-welded cruciform joints, the actual root gap should be taken as the initial crack. It is convenient to disregard the threshold properties. Later, the obtained fatigue cycles may be converted into a FAT class, of which the S–N curve will be used further on.

$$FAT = \Delta\sigma_{\text{applied}} \cdot \sqrt[m]{\frac{N}{2 \times 10^6}}$$

8.3 Fatigue Assessment by Crack Propagation

$$\Delta K_{i,s,d} = \Delta K_{i,s,k} \cdot \gamma_F$$

The fatigue action represented by the design spectrum of SIF ranges is verified by the material resistance design parameters against crack propagation

$$C_{0,d} = C_{0,k} \cdot \gamma_M = C_{0,k} \cdot \Gamma^M$$

$$\frac{da}{dN} = C_0 \cdot \Delta K^m \quad \text{if } \Delta K < \Delta K_{\text{th}} \text{ then } \frac{da}{dN} = 0$$

$$\Delta K_{\text{th},d} = \frac{\Delta K_{\text{th},k}}{\gamma_M}$$

using the "Paris–Erdogan" power law
where

a Crack size
N Number of cycles
ΔK Stress intensity factor range
ΔK_{th} Threshold value of stress intensity factor range below which no crack propagation is assumed
C_0, m Material constants
γ_F, γ_M Partial safety factors

For applied SIFs, which are high compared with the fracture toughness of the material, K_c, an acceleration of crack propagation will occur. In these cases, the following extension of the "Paris" power law of crack propagation is recommended. In the absence of an accurate value of the fracture toughness, a conservative estimate should be made.

$$\frac{da}{dN} = \frac{C_0 \cdot \Delta K^m}{(1-R) - \frac{\Delta K}{K_{mat}}}$$

where

K_{mat} Fracture toughness
R Stress ratio

The fatigue life N is determined by integration starting from an initial crack parameter a_i to a final one a_f. The calculated number of life cycles N must be greater or equal to the required number of life cycles.

The same formulae apply for a crack growth calculation in a **c**-direction, if that was required by the selected procedure.

In general, the integration has to be carried out numerically. The increment for one cycle is

$$da = C_{0,d} \cdot \Delta K_{a,d} \quad \text{if } \Delta K_{a,d} < K_{th,d} \text{ else } da = 0$$
$$dc = C_{0,d} \cdot \Delta K_{c,d} \quad \text{if } \Delta K_{c,d} < K_{th,d} \text{ else } dc = 0$$

It is recommended that a continuous spectrum is subdivided into an adequate number of stress range blocks, e.g., 8 or 10 blocks, and that the integration is performed block-wise by summing the increments of a and the number of cycles of the blocks. The entire size of the spectrum in terms of cycles should be adjusted by multiplying the block cycles by an appropriate factor in order to ensure at least 20 loops over the whole spectrum in the integration procedure. If the sequence of loading is not known, the highest stresses in spectrum should be processed first.

When using weight functions, the integration of the power law of crack propagation has to be performed over the implicit integral of the weight function.

$$N = \int_{x=0}^{x=a_f} \frac{C_0 \cdot \mathrm{d}x}{\Delta K^m} = \int_{a=0}^{a=a_f} \frac{C_0 \cdot \mathrm{d}x}{\left[\int_{x=0}^{x=a_i} \Delta\sigma(x) \cdot h(x,a) \cdot \mathrm{d}x\right]^m}$$

8.4 Material Parameters for Crack Propagation

The resistance of a material against cyclic crack propagation is characterized by the material parameters of the "Paris–Erdogan" power law of crack propagation

$$\frac{\mathrm{d}a}{\mathrm{d}N} = C_0 \cdot \Delta K^m \quad \text{if } \Delta K < \Delta K_{\mathrm{th}} \text{ then } \frac{\mathrm{d}a}{\mathrm{d}N} = 0$$

where the material parameters are

C_0 Constant of the power law
m Exponent of the power law
ΔK Range of cyclic stress intensity factor
ΔK_{th} Threshold value of stress intensity, under which no crack propagation is assumed
R Stress ratio, taking all stresses including residual stresses into account

In the absence of specified or measured material parameters, the values given below are recommended, see Tables 8.1 and 8.2. They are characteristic values, which typically mean that the computed fatigue life corresponds to a 95 % survival probability.

For elevated temperatures other than room temperature or for metallic materials other than steel, the crack propagation parameters vary with the modulus of elasticity E and may be determined accordingly.

$$C = C_{0,\mathrm{steel}} \cdot \left(\frac{E_{\mathrm{steel}}}{E}\right)^m \tag{8.1}$$

$$\Delta K_{\mathrm{th}} = \Delta K_{\mathrm{th,steel}} \cdot \left(\frac{E}{E_{\mathrm{steel}}}\right) \tag{8.2}$$

Table 8.1 Parameters of the Paris power law and threshold data for steel

Units	Paris power law parameters	Threshold values ΔK_{th}			
		$R \geq 0.5$	$0 \leq R \leq 0.5$	$R < 0$	Surface crack depth <1 mm
K (N mm$^{-3/2}$) $\mathrm{d}a/\mathrm{d}N$ (mm/cycle)	$C_0 = 5.21 \times 10^{-13}$ $m = 3.0$	63	$170–214 \cdot R$	170	≤63
K (MPa$\sqrt{m}$) $\mathrm{d}a/\mathrm{d}N$ (m/cycle)	$C_0 = 1.65 \times 10^{-11}$ $m = 3.0$	2.0	$5.4–6.8 \cdot R$	5.4	≤2.0

Table 8.2 Parameters of the Paris power law and threshold data for aluminum

Units	Paris power law parameters	Threshold values ΔK_{th}			
		$R \geq 0.5$	$0 \leq R \leq 0.5$	$R < 0$	Surface crack depth <1 mm
K (N mm$^{-3/2}$) da/dN (mm/cycle)	$C_0 = 1.41 \times 10^{-11}$ m = 3.0	21	56.7–72.3 · R	56.7	≤21
K (MPa$\sqrt{m}$) da/dN (m/cycle)	$C_0 = 4.46 \times 10^{-10}$ m = 3.0	0.7	1.8–2.3 · R	1.8	≤0.7

8.5 Dimensions of Cracks

Cracks or crack-like defects found in work shop may have various sizes and shapes. In order to fit them into the fracture mechanics world, they need to be assessed in some simplified way. This is described in Table 8.3.

Table 8.3 Dimensions for assessment of crack-like imperfections (example)

Idealizations and dimensions of crack-like imperfection for fracture mechanics assessment procedure (t = wall thickness)

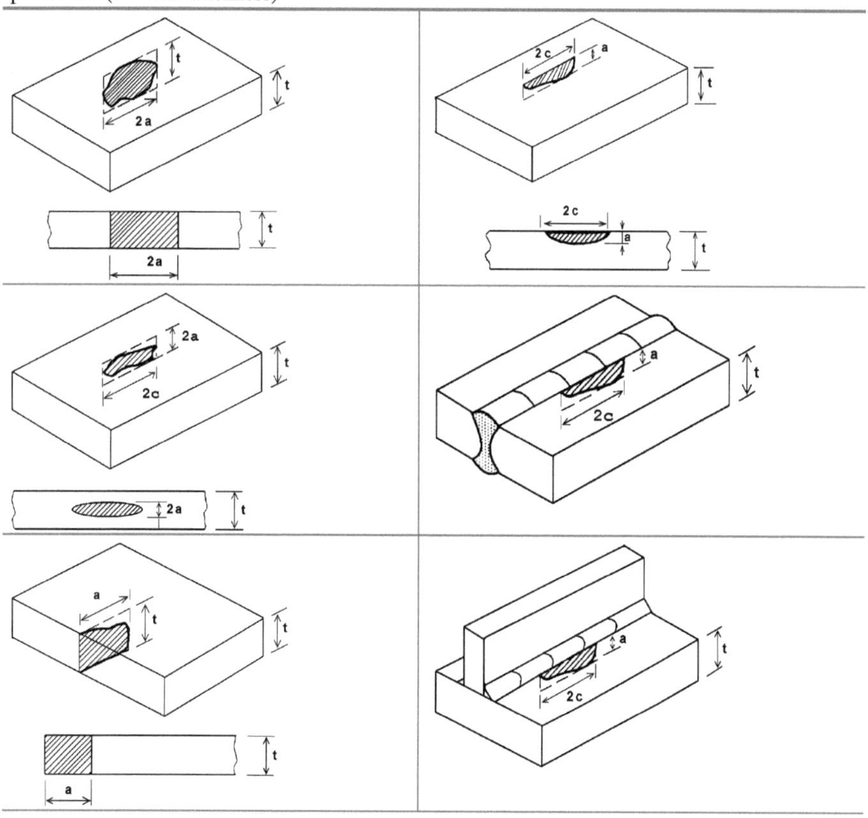

Adjacent cracks may interact and behave like a single large one. The interaction between adjacent cracks should be checked according to an interaction criterion.

There are different interaction criteria, and in consequence no strict recommendation can be given. It is recommended to proceed according to an accepted code, e.g. Ref. [4] in Chap. 6.

8.6 Formulae for Stress Intensity Factors

SIF formulae may be taken from literature, see Refs. [1–8]. The formulae given below address only some of the cases relevant to welded joints. They are given as a base for two examples, which follows below.

8.6.1 *Standard Solutions*

See Table 8.4

Table 8.4 Stress intensity factors

Surface cracks under membrane stress	
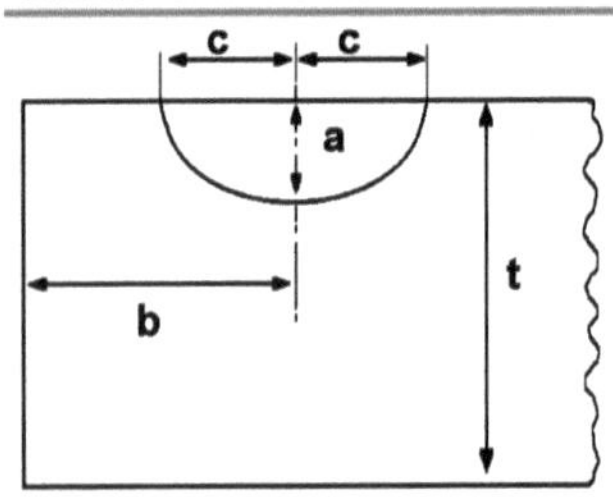 **b = distance to nearest edge**	The formula for the stress intensity factor K_1 is valid for $a/c < 1$, for more details see Ref. [2]
$K_1 = \sigma \sqrt{(\pi \cdot a/Q)} \cdot F_s$	
$Q = 1 + 1.464\ (a/c)^{1.65}$	
$F_s = [M_1 + M_2 \cdot (a/t)^2 + M_3 \cdot (a/t)^4] \cdot g \cdot f \cdot f_w$	
$M_1 = 1.13 - 0.09\ (a/c)$	
$M_2 = -0.54 + 0.89/(0.2 + a/c)$	
$M_3 = 0.5 - 1/(0.65 + a/c) + 14\ (1 - a/c)^{24}$	
$f_w = [\sec(\pi \cdot c \sqrt{(a/t)}/(2 \cdot b))]^{1/2}$	
g and f are dependent on direction	
"a"-direction: $g = 1$ $f = 1$	
"c"-direction: $g = 1 + [0.1 + 0.35\ (a/t)^2]$	
$f = \sqrt{(a/c)}$	
Embedded cracks under membrane stress	

(continued)

Table 8.4 (continued)

Surface cracks under membrane stress	
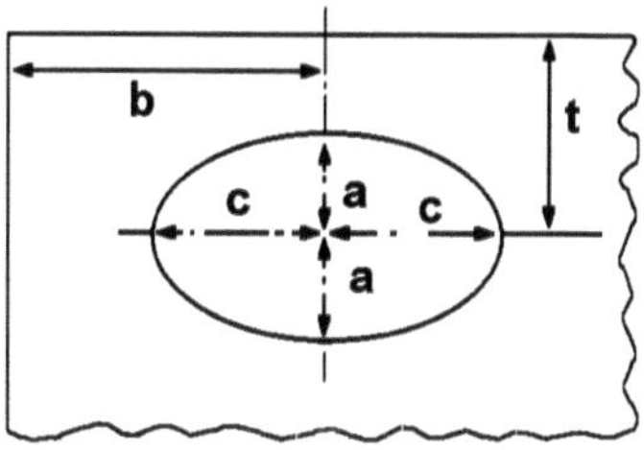 **t = distance to nearest surface**	The formula for the stress intensity factor K_1 is valid for $a/c < 1$, for more details see Ref. [2]
K_1, Q, F_s, f_w as given before for surface cracks, but	
$M_1 = 1$	
$M_2 = 0.05/(0.11 + (a/c)^{3/2})$	
$M_3 = 0.29/(0.23 + (a/c)^{3/2})$	
g and f are dependent on direction	
"a"-direction: $g = 1 \quad f = 1$	
"c"-direction: $g = 1 - (a/t)^4/(1 + 4a/c)$ $f = \sqrt{(a/c)}$	
Root gap crack in a fillet-welded cruciform joint	
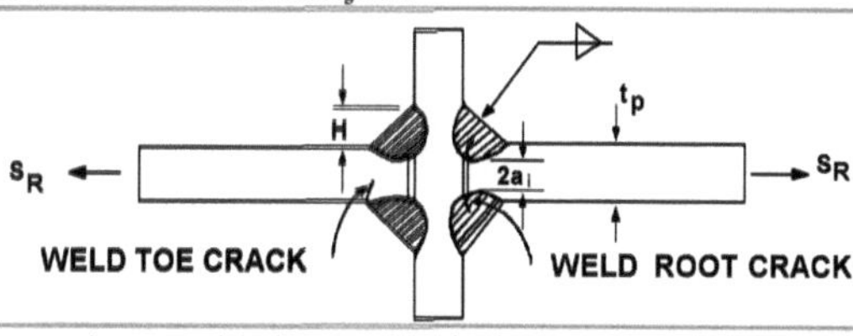 	The formula for the stress intensity factor K is valid for H/t from 0.2 to 1.2 and for a/w from 0.0 to 0.7. For more details see Ref. [5]
$K = \frac{\sigma(A_1 + A_2 \cdot a/w)\sqrt{(\pi \cdot a \cdot \sec(\pi \cdot a/2w))}}{1 + 2 \cdot H/t}$	
where $w = H + t/2$	
σ = nominal stress range in the longitudinal plates	
and with $x = H/t$	
$A_1 = 0.528 + 3.287 \cdot x - 4.361 \cdot x^2 + 3.696 \cdot x^3 - 1.875 \cdot x^4 + 0.415 \cdot x^5$	
$A_2 = 0.218 + 2.717 \cdot x - 10.171 \cdot x^2 + 13.122 \cdot x^3 - 7.755 \cdot x^4 + 1.783 \cdot x^5$	

8.6.2 Solutions for Magnification Function Mk

Parametric formulae for M_k functions have been established for a variety of welded joints [7, 8].

Below one formula is given, where the 3-dimensional effects are included for a semicircular weld toe crack. The M_k-values are given and to get the stress intensity values, the Y-factors also need to be computed, see Table 8.2, where the Y-factor can be identified as $F_s/\sqrt{Q}$ in formula of K_1.

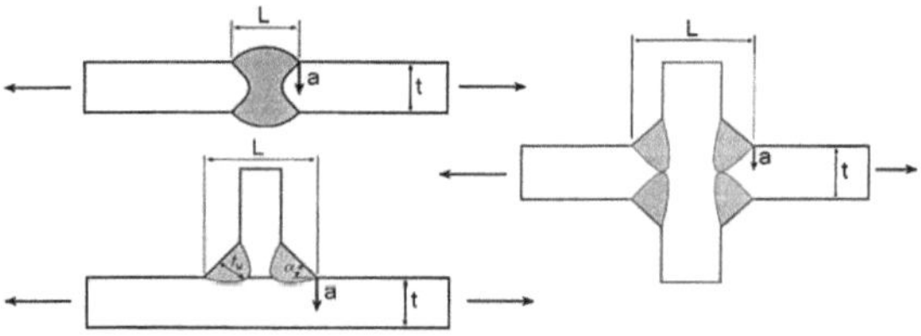

Fig. 8.3 Relevant dimensions for different joint types

This 3-dimensional Mk-solution was published by Bowness and Lee [12, 13], where the fitted formulae are valid for membrane stress and a weld toe angle of 45° and (Fig. 8.3):

$$0.005 < a/t < 1.0$$
$$0.1 < a/c < 1.0$$
$$0.5 < L/t < 2.75 \quad \text{if } L/t > 2.75 \text{ then } L/t = 2.75$$

Deepest point

$$g_1 = -1.0343 * (a/c) \wedge 2 - 0.1567 * (a/c) + 1.3409$$
$$g_2 = 1.3218 * (a/c) \wedge -0.61153$$
$$g_3 = -0.87238 * (a/c) + 1.2788$$
$$g_4 = -0.46190 * (a/c) \wedge 3 + 0.6709 * (a/c) \wedge 2 - 0.37571 * (a/c) + 4.6511$$
$$f_1 = 0.43358 * (a/t) \wedge (g_1 + (g_2 * (a/t)) \wedge g_3) + 0.93163 * \exp((a/t) \wedge -0.050966) + g_4$$
$$f_2 = -0.21521 * (1 - (a/t)) \wedge 176.4199 + 2.8141 * (a/t) \wedge (-0.1074 * (a/t))$$
$$g_5 = -0.015647 * (L/t) \wedge 3 + 0.09889 * (L/t) \wedge 2 - 0.17180 * (L/t) - 0.24587$$
$$g_6 = -0.20136 * (L/t) \wedge 2 + 0.93311 * (L/t) - 0.41496$$
$$g_7 = 0.20188 * (L/t) \wedge 2 - 0.97857 * (L/t) + 0.068225$$
$$g_8 = -0.027338 * (L/t) \wedge 2 + 0.12551 * (L/t) - 11.281$$
$$f_3 = 0.33994 * (a/t) \wedge g_5 + 1.9493 * (a/t) \wedge 0.23003 + (g_6 * (a/t) \wedge 2 + g_7 * (a/t) + g_8)$$

$$M_{ka} = f_1 + f_2 + f_3 \quad \text{if } M_{ka} < 1 \text{ then } M_{ka} = 1$$

Surface point

$$g_1 = 0.0078157 * c/a \wedge 2 - 0.070664 * c/a + 1.8508$$
$$g_2 = -0.000054546 * (L/t) \wedge 2 + 0.00013651 * (L/t) - 0.00047844$$
$$g_3 = 0.00049192 * (L/t) \wedge 2 - 0.0013595 * (L/t) + 0.011400$$
$$g_4 = 0.0071654 * (L/t) \wedge 2 - 0.033399 * (L/t) - 0.25064$$
$$g_5 = -0.018640 * c/a \wedge 2 + 0.24311 * c/a - 1.7644$$
$$g_6 = -0.001671 * (L/t) \wedge 2 + 0.0090620 * (L/t) - 0.016479$$
$$g_7 = -0.0031615 * (L/t) \wedge 2 - 0.010944 * (L/t) + 0.13967$$

$g_8 = -0.045206 * (L/t) \wedge 3 + 0.32380 * (L/t) \wedge 2 - 0.68935 * (L/t) + 1.4954$
$f_1 = g_1 * (a/t) \wedge (g_2 * c/a \wedge 2 + g_3 * c/a + g_4) + g_5 * (1 - (a/t)) \wedge (g_6 * c/a \wedge 2 + g_7 * c/a + g_8)$
$g_9 = -0.25473 * (a/c) \wedge 2 + 0.40928 * (a/c) + 0.0021892$
$g_{10} = 37.423 * (a/c) \wedge 2 - 15.741 * (a/c) + 64.903$
$f_2 = (-0.28639 * (a/c) \wedge 2 + 0.35411 * (a/c) + 1.643) * (a/t) \wedge g_9 + 0.27449 * (1 - (a/t)) \wedge g_{10}$
$g_{11} = -0.10553 * (L/t) \wedge 3 + 0.59894 * (L/t) \wedge 2 - 1.0942 * (L/t) - 1.2650$
$g_{12} = 0.043891 * (L/t) \wedge 3 - 0.24898 * (L/t) \wedge 2 + 0.44732 * (L/t) + 0.60136$
$g_{13} = -0.011411 * (a/c) \wedge 2 + 0.004369 * (a/c) + 0.51732$
$f_3 = g_{11} * (a/t) \wedge 0.75429 + g_{12} * \exp((a/t) \wedge g_{13})$

$$M_{kc} = f_1 * f_2 * f_3 \quad \text{if } M_{kc} < 1 \text{ then } M_{kc} = 1$$

8.6.3 *Examples of a Fracture Mechanics Assessment*

Below two examples are given, where linear fracture mechanics is being used to assess the fatigue life in a welded joint. The first example describes a toe crack found in work shop, where the M_k- and *Y*-factors are used. The second describes an ordinary fillet weld having a partial penetration and where the weld is load-carrying, thus leading to a critical weld root side. Here, there exists a direct formula for the stress intensity at the weld root. Both cases are compared with other methods for validation purposes. For deeper studies, Refs. [14, 17, 18, 20–42] may be used.

8.6.3.1 Crack at the Toe of a Fillet Weld of a Cruciform Joint

A crack was detected in a weld toe connection a tensile bar and a transverse stiffener. The residual life cycles had to be calculated, see Fig. 8.4.

The detected crack had the following dimensions: Depth a = 2 mm, length $2c$ = 20 mm. An acceptable final crack could be 1/2 wall thickness; thus, final depth

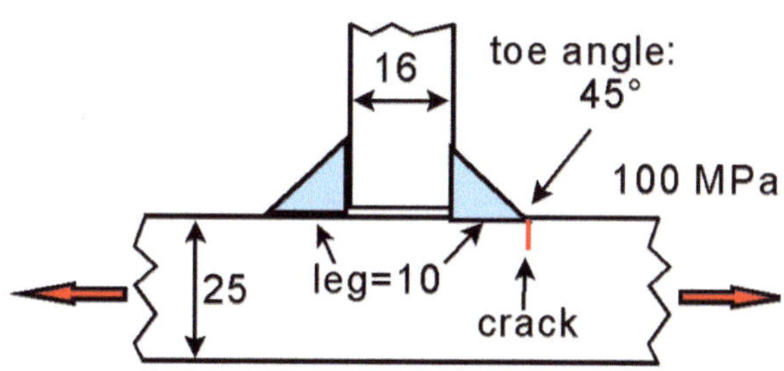

Fig. 8.4 Geometry of weld toe problem

(a) is 12.5 mm. How many cycles could be expected for a crack to propagate from the initial to the final crack?

Correction functions for a surface crack (Y_a- and Y_c-factors) were taken from Newman and Raju: ASTM STP 791 1983, pp. I-238–I-265. The aspect ratio was calculated by incrementing a and c according to the Newman–Raju formulae, and M_{ka}- and M_{kc}-functions were taken from Bowness and Lee, Int. J. Fatigue 22(2000) pp. 369–387, Refs. [11, 12]. Stress intensities were computed as follows (see Sect. 8.6):

$$\mathrm{d}K = \Delta\sigma * Y * M_k * \sqrt{(\pi\, a)} \quad \text{for } a \text{ and } c\text{-directions respectively}$$

The constants of the Paris–Erdogan power law of crack propagation are as follows: $C_0 = 1.65\mathrm{e}{-11}$ $m = 3$ when units [MPa] and [m/cycle] are used. Note that these numbers are characteristic values implying a certain safety margin.

The calculation gives the data given in Table 8.5, see also Figs. 8.5 and 8.6. Note that steps used in the analysis must be smaller than indicated in Table 8.5, where only a few steps are shown.

A stress range in plate of $\Delta\sigma = 100$ MPa results in 255890 cycles, corresponding to a fatigue class of 50 MPa at 2 million cycles. While the crack propagated down into 12.5 mm wall thickness, it has spread out at the surface from tip to tip to $2 \cdot \mathrm{c} = 2 \cdot 27 = 54$ mm.

A comparison of the results above using a FEM solution (indicated by point-markers in Fig. 8.5) confirms the stress intensity for the deepest point (a): FE gives dK_a = 9.7 while the formulas used give dK_a = 8.9 [MPa$\sqrt{\text{m}}$]. However, for the surface point (c), there is a difference: FE gives dK_c = 7.2 while the formulas give dK_c = 11.0 [MPa$\sqrt{\text{m}}$], see model in Fig. 8.7.

Table 8.5 Computed parameters and fatigue life

a (mm)	c (mm)	Mk_a (–)	Mk_c (–)	Y_a (–)	Y_c (–)	dK_a (–) [MPaV(m)]	dK_c [MPaV(m)]	N (cycles)
2	10.0	1.045	2.640	1.069	0.527	8.9	11.0	0
2.5	11.0	1.000	2.423	1.060	0.557	9.4	12.0	40719
3	12.0	1.000	2.261	1.053	0.581	10.2	12.8	73748
4	13.9	1.000	2.028	1.043	0.621	11.7	14.1	121013
5	15.6	1.000	1.869	1.036	0.654	13.0	15.3	153894
6	17.2	1.000	1.754	1.033	0.684	14.2	16.5	178429
7	18.7	1.000	1.668	1.033	0.712	15.3	17.6	197564
8	20.2	1.000	1.603	1.035	0.739	16.4	18.8	212940
9	21.7	1.000	1.553	1.039	0.766	17.5	20.0	225560
10	23.2	1.000	1.513	1.044	0.792	18.5	21.2	236082
11	24.8	1.000	1.482	1.052	0.819	19.6	22.6	244961
12	26.3	1.000	1.457	1.061	0.846	20.6	23.9	252523
12.5	27.1	1.000	1.446	1.066	0.860	21.2	24.8	255890

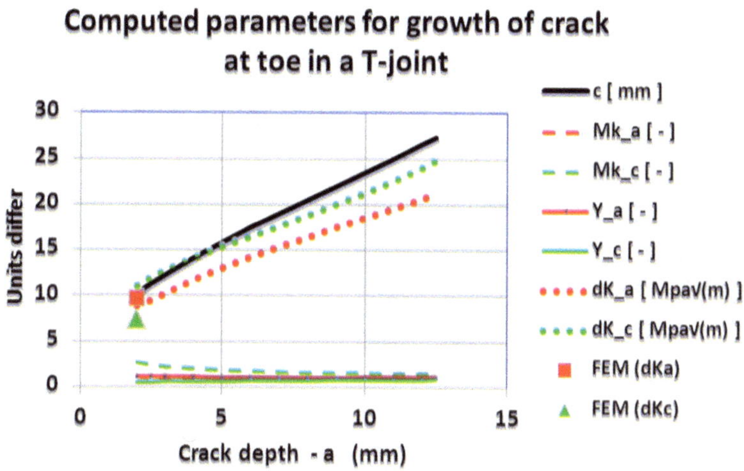

Fig. 8.5 Parameters from Table 8.5 (units on *Y*-axis is shown in legend)

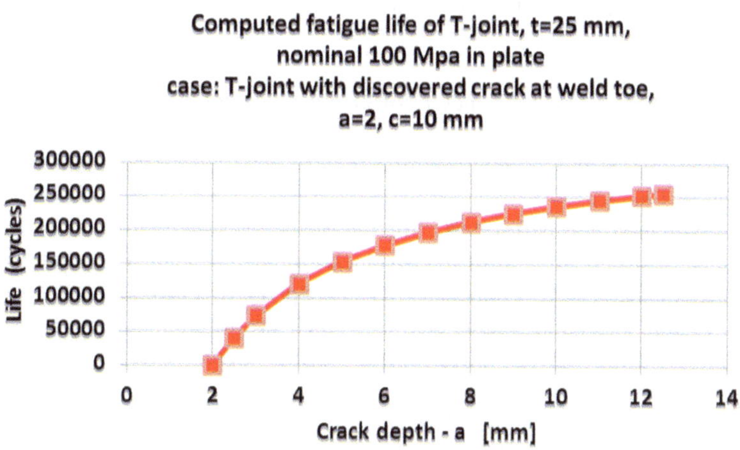

Fig. 8.6 Life (cycles) along crack growth, note that "*a*" trends to go to infinity after *t*/2 indicating that the fatigue life is near over

The difference between the formulas and the FE solution is not quite explained. The FE-model is built as a cruciform joint, which might have a slightly different behavior compared to the T-joint. However, if a true T-joint is modeled without any particular supports, then d*K_a* fits even better, but the difference in d*K_c* stays un-changed and one problem with this model is that there is a clear bending behavior which do not fit into a T-joint with a tension load.

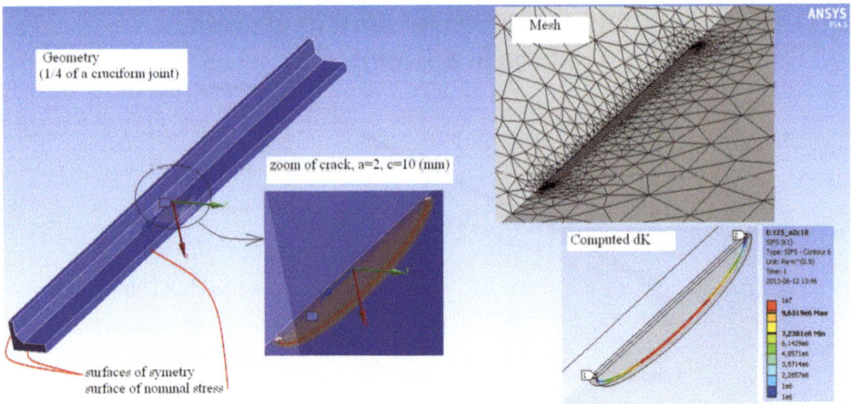

Fig. 8.7 FEM solution of starting crack size (a = 2, c = 10). dK_a = 9.7 and dK_c = 7.2

So overall, the fatigue life will probably be similar for both cases of FEM or formulas. The main difference would probably be visible as a difference in crack growth in the c-direction. This was not investigated.

8.6.3.2 Weld with Partial Penetration (Root Gap) in a Cruciform Joint

A cruciform joint with partial penetration shall be assessed for its fatigue properties as shown in Fig. 8.8.

The calculation was performed using the correction function of Frank K.H. and Fisher J.W.: Fatigue strength of fillet-welded cruciform joints. J. of the Structural Div., Proc. of the ASCE, Volume 105 (1979) pp. 1727–1740, see Table 8.4.

The fracture mechanics parameters for crack propagation are C_0 = 1.65e−11 (units in N and m) and m = 3. Here, the validity range has to be considered (a/w < 0.7). The initial crack is given by the weld face gap of tip to tip of 10 mm. The initial crack parameter is then 1/2 of that, thus a = 5 mm. The end of the validity range at 16 mm was taken as the final crack. The constant parameters among the formulas are computed to Table 8.6.

Stepwise increasing crack "a" from 5 to 16 mm will now give the following results (note that steps used in the analysis must be smaller than indicated, only a few steps are shown), see Table 8.7.

Having 100 MPa stress in the plate will thus result in a life of 185145 cycles. This can also be recalculated to a 2 million stress range corresponding to a stress level of 45 MPa (FAT 45), related to nominal stress in plate. In relation to the weld throat this corresponds to 39 MPa (resulting in FAT 36).

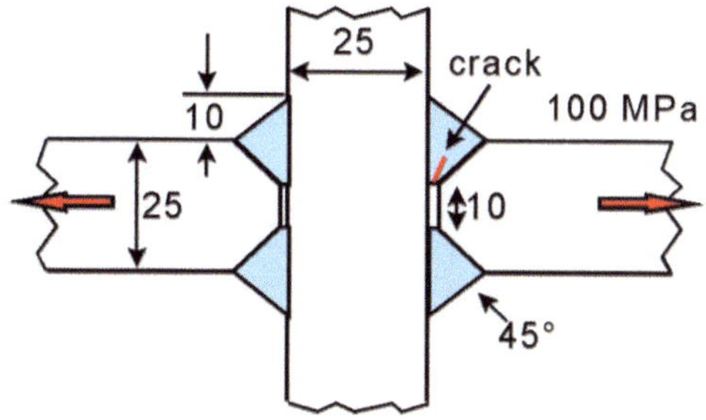

Fig. 8.8 Geometry of weld root problem

Table 8.6 Value of some parameters

Denominator in *K*	*A*1	*A*2	*w* (mm)	*x*
1.8	1.338	0.337	22.5	0.4

Table 8.7 Computed parameters and fatigue life

a (mm)	Numerator in *K*	*K* [MPa sq. root (m)]	*N* (cycles)
5	577.6	10.15	0
5.5	613.1	10.77	27009
6	648.5	11.39	49688
7	720.0	12.65	85341
8	793.5	13.94	111658
9	870.6	15.29	131443
10	952.7	16.74	146481
11	1041.5	18.30	157977
12	1139.1	20.01	166773
13	1248.2	21.93	173482
14	1372.4	24.11	178560
15	1516.9	26.65	182357
16	1689.2	29.68	185145

Using the effective notch method for this case, see Fig. 8.9, results in a computed notch stress of 481 MPa, and using FAT 225 this implies a computed fatigue life of 204712 cycles, approximately 10 % over the fracture mechanics results above, thus well in agreement.

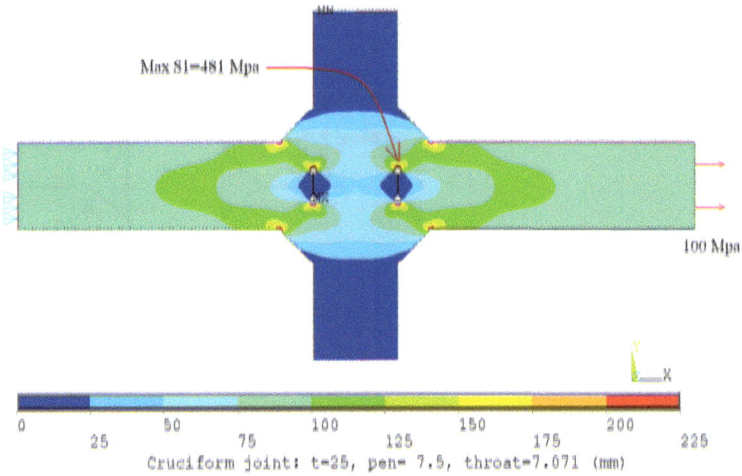

Fig. 8.9 FEM solution using the effective notch method. Toe stress is around 80 % of the root and thus not the critical point

8.7 Computation of Results Using Design of Experiments Theory

One way to make studies over how geometry parameters and imperfections influence the fatigue behavior of a weld is to use design of experiments (DoE). This method can be used not only in real performed physical testing, it can also be used within analysis, where simulations replace the tests. The most suitable analysis method to use for welds is the effective notch method, where many of the different weld parameters can be taken into account and studied. This makes it possible to perform "full tests" so that all combinations of the parameters are computed and where one can regard parameters with small effect on the result as scatter. Parameters having an effect greater than say one standard deviation from mean can then be regarded as the important ones. The example shown here has been done using a 2-level DoE, where the parameters are varied at 2 levels: high and low. It is suitable to set these 2 levels on each side of a typical mean value for each parameter studied; as an example, if throat size typically is 5 mm, then low level might be set to 4 and high level to 6 mm. The assumption is then that all variations of throat sizes from 4 to 6 mm are covered (linear behavior assumed).

8.7.1 *Butt Welded from 1 Side Only, Flexible Boundary Conditions*

A butt welded from only one side, see Fig. 8.10, will most of the times have the weak point on the root (back) side of the weld, since there is a big risk of having defects or lack of full penetration here. The geometry chosen in this study has a width of the weld = thickness of the plate with rather flexible boundary conditions in the sense that bending is allowed. Six parameters are varied (low and high) (giving $2^6 = 64$ different simulations):

Undercut, u	0.1–1 mm
Thickness, t	8–12 mm
Toe radius, R (FEM)	1–2 mm
Root defect, rd	0.1–1 mm
S-measure, s	$(t - \text{rd})$
Angle, α	10°–30°

The result of such a study is presented in Fig. 8.11, where the Y-axis gives the computed stress responses in the weld toe and root, respectively, expressed as a percentage of 225 MPa with an applied nominal tension load = 100 MPa. If the computed stress is >0 (column up), the implication is that an increase in this parameter level gives arise to an increase in stress response and vice versa. The results indicate that with the chosen parameter levels, the lack of penetration is the most important one for the root, followed by the undercut size for the toe. Another conclusion is that the angle has a very low influence, which is interesting to realize having in mind that some weld quality rules put (un-needed) attention to this angle.

8.7.2 *Butt Welded from 2 Sides, Symmetric Weld*

A close-related case to the one in Sect. 8.7.1 is when a butt joint is welded from both sides with symmetric geometry, which means that any lack of penetration will be positioned in the middle of the plate, see Fig. 8.12.

Parameters for this case are the same as for the 1-sided butt weld apart from the thickness. Since this is a 2-sided weld, there is a reason to assume bigger thicknesses (10–20 mm), and also the root defect (rd) will now be given by the s-measure = $(t - \text{rd})/2$. The results of this study indicate the same conclusions as for

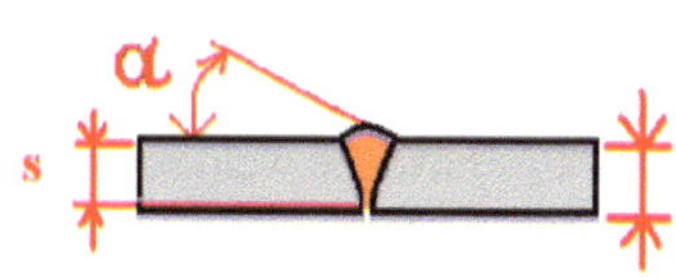

Fig. 8.10 Butt joint

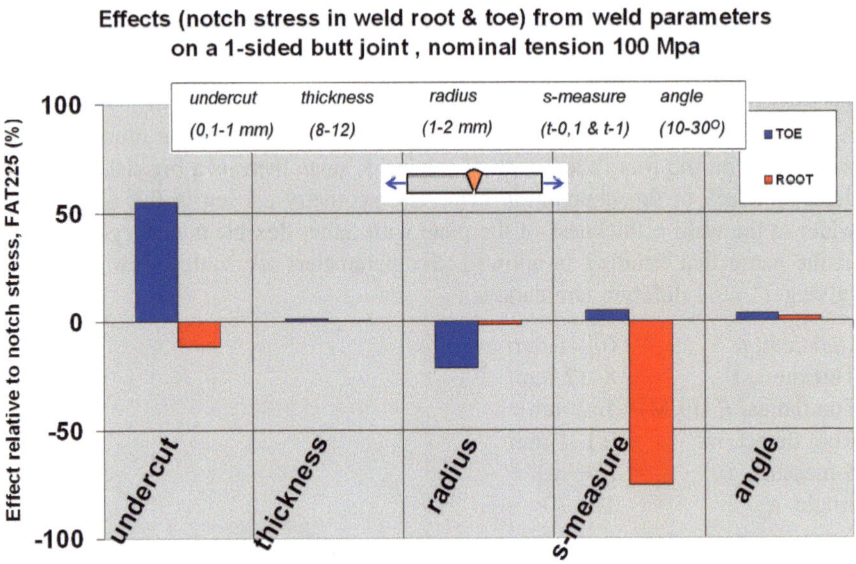

Fig. 8.11 Computed relative effects for a 1-s butt weld in tension, nominal 100 MPa

Fig. 8.12 2-sided butt weld

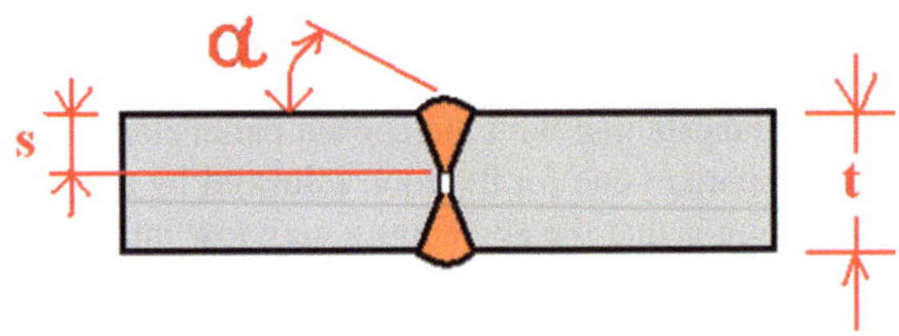

the 1-sided butt weld that under the chosen parameter levels, the lack of penetration is the most important one for the root (the bigger s-measure the lower stress at the root), followed by the undercut size for the toe, see Fig. 8.13, even though the influence from the undercut is smaller for the 2-sided butt weld compared to the 1-sided joint, probably depending on the fact that the 1-sided butt joint allows some bending even for pure tension, see Fig. 8.11 and the boundary conditions for this case. One can also see that the angle has also here a very low influence similar to the 1-side welded butt joint.

8.7.3 Load-Carrying Cruciform Joint

A cruciform joint where the load passes through the weld, see Fig. 8.14, will in most cases have the weld root (weld back side) as the critical point. This is reflected in the standards by setting a FAT value of 36 or 40 MPa based on the throat size.

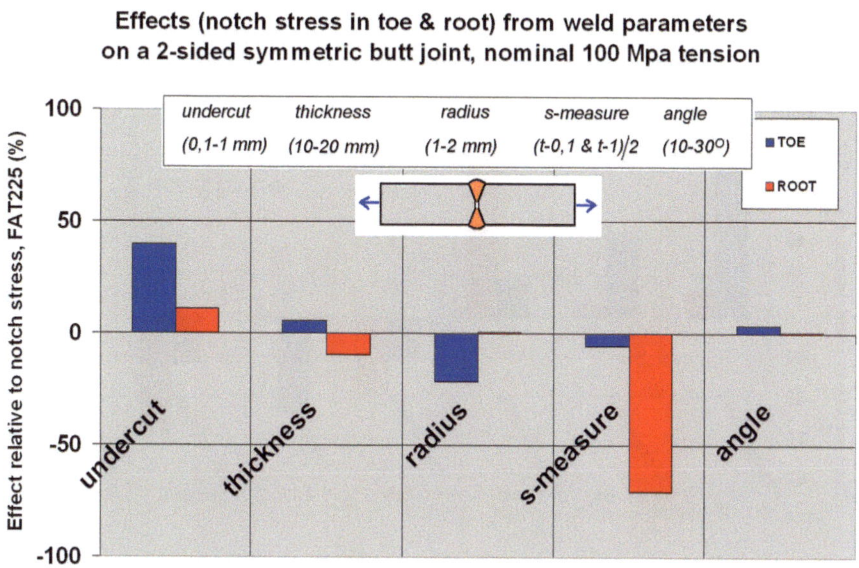

Fig. 8.13 Computed relative effects for a 2-s butt weld in tension, nominal 100 MPa

Fig. 8.14 Fillet joint

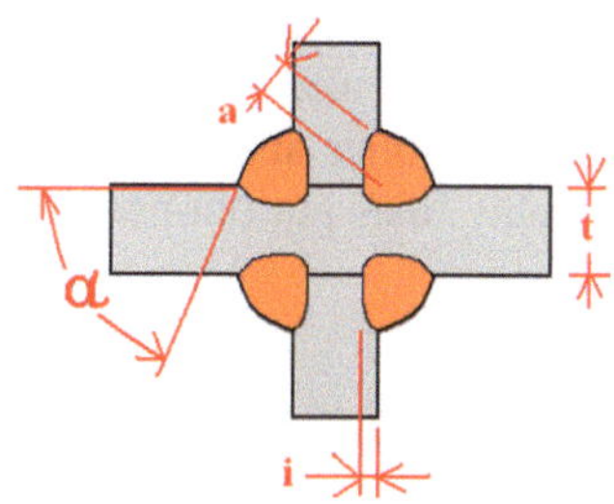

The 7 parameters varied in this example are (giving $2^7 = 128$ computer simulations):

Undercut, *u*	0.1–1 mm
Thickness, *t*	8–12 mm
Toe radius, *R* (FEM)	1–2 mm
Throat size, *a*	4–6 mm
Penetration, *i*	1–3 mm
Misalignment	0.1–1.5 mm
Angle, *α*	30°–60°

The result of such a study indicates that with the chosen parameter levels, the weld toe side is affected by misalignment and undercut for increased stress and toe

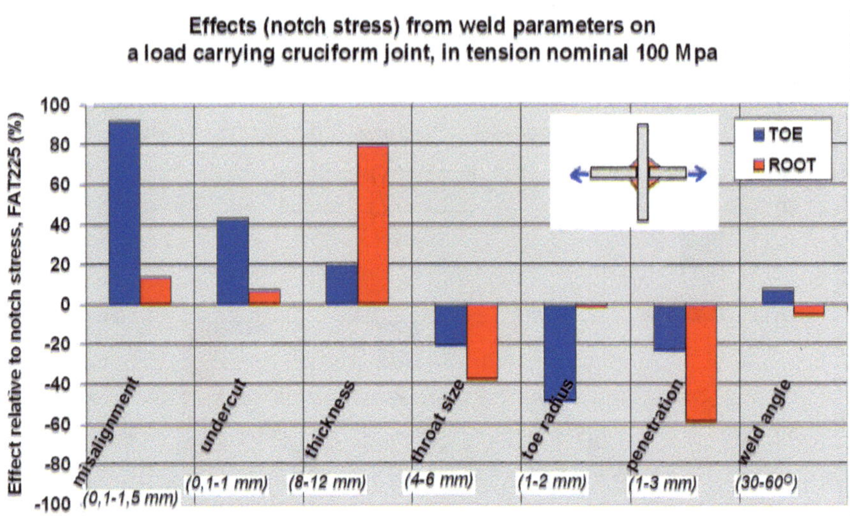

Fig. 8.15 Computed effects for a load-carrying fillet weld in tension, nominal 100 MPa

radius for decreased stress. The weld root is affected mostly by thickness for increase of stress while penetration and throat size tends to decrease the stress, see Fig. 8.15.

One can also see that the angle has a very low influence well in agreement with the butt joints above. Again this is interesting to notice having in mind that many quality rules put (un-needed) attention to this parameter as a quality assurance.

8.7.4 *Non-load-Carrying Cruciform Joint*

A non-load-carrying cruciform joint, where the load is going through the main plate only passing aside of the weld, shows quite another behavior in comparison with a load-carrying cruciform joint. Typical is that the parameters play a much smaller role compared to a load-carrying fillet weld and also that the weld toe at the main plate will now be critical instead of the weld root. Looking at the FAT levels for this joint, one can find values from 63 to 80 MPa (for the weld toe) depending on the case at hand. This means that penetration and misalignment are more or less un-important, while an undercut (increases the stress) and the toe radius (decreases the stress) have a big influence on the weld toe near the main plate, see Fig. 8.16 and these are more or less the only parameters which have an effect. One can also see that the impact from the toe radius is now smaller for the non-load-carrying fillet joint, approximately 30 % compared to 50 % for the load-carrying cruciform joint. This depends on the fact that the K_t-factor at the weld toe is higher for a load-carrying case than for the non-load-carrying case.

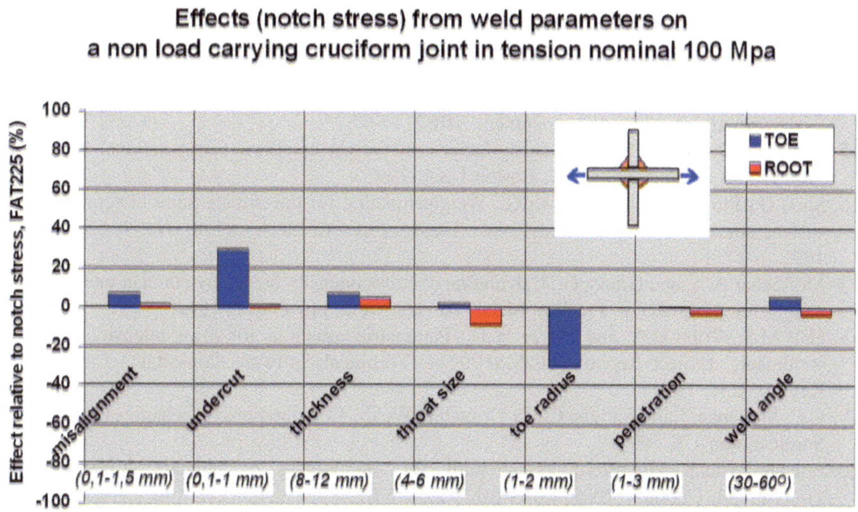

Fig. 8.16 Computed effects for a non-load-carrying fillet weld in tension, nominal 100 MPa

References

1. Murakami Y. Stress Intensity Factors Handbook Pergamon Press, Oxford U.K. 1987
2. Newman J.C. and Raju I.S. Stress intensity factor equations for cracks in three-dimensional finite bodies. ASTM STP 791 1983, pp. I-238 - I-265
3. Newman J.C. and Raju I.S. Stress intensity factors for internal surface cracks in cylindrical pressure vessels. Journal of Pressure Vessel Technology, 102 (1980), pp. 342-346.
4. Newman J.C. and Raju I.S. An empirical stress intensity factor equation for the surface crack. Engineering Fracture Mechanics, Vol 15. 1981, No 1-2, pp. 185-192
5. Frank K.H. and Fisher J.W. Fatigue strength of fillet welded cruciform joints. J. of the Structural Div., Proc. of the ASCE, Vol 105 (1979) pp. 1727-1740
6. Folias E.S. Axial crack in pressurized cylindrical shell. Int. J. of Fracture Mechanics, vol 1 (1965) No. 2, pp 104
7. Hobbacher A. Stress intensity factors of welded joints. Engineering Fracture Mechanics, Vol 46 (1993), no 2, pp. 173-182, and Vol 49 (1994), no 2, p. 323
8. Maddox S.J. and Andrews R.M. Stress intensity factors for weld toe cracks, in 'Localized Damage Computer Aided Assessment and Control'. Aliabadi M.H., Brebbia C.A. and Cartwright D.J. (Editors). Computational Mechanics Publications, Southamton, ISBN 1 853 12 070 7, co-published with Springer-Verlag, Heidelberg, ISBN 3 540 527 17 6, 1990
9. Albrecht P. And Yamada K. Rapid calculation of stress intensity factors. J. Struct. Div. ASCE, 1977, 103(ST2), 377-389
10. Pang H.L.J. A review of stress intensity factors for semi-elliptical surface crack in a plate and fillet welded joint. The Welding Institute, Abington, Cambridge UK, TWI Report 426/1990, IIW doc. XIII-1433-91
11. Bowness D. and Lee M.M.K.: Stress intensity factor solutions for semi-elliptical weld-toe cracks in T-butt geometries. Fatigue Fract. Engg. Mater. Struct. Vol. 19, No. 6, pp 787-797, 1996.
12. Bowness D. and Lee M.M.K.: Prediction of weld toe magnification factors for semi-elliptical cracks in T-but joints. Int. J. Fatigue, 22 (5), 389-396, 2000.

13. Engesvik K.M.:Analysis of uncertainties in the fatigue capacity of welded joints, Doctoral Thesis, Division of Marine Structures, University of Trondheim, Norwegian Institute of Technology, Trondheim Norway, 1981
14. Nykänen T., Marquis G. and Björk T.: Simplified assessment of weld quality for fatigue loaded cruciform joints. IIW document XIII-2177-07
15. Fett T. and Munz D.: Stress intensity factors and weight functions. Computational Mechanics Publications, Southampton UK, Boston USA, 1997
16. Shen G., Plumtree A. and Glinka G.: Weight function for the surface point of semi elliptical surfece crack in a finite thickness plate. Engng. Fracture Mech. vol 40, No. 1, pp 167-176, 1991.
17. Moftakhar A.A. and Glinka G.: Calculation of stress intensity factors by efficient integration of weight functions. Engg. Fracture Mech. vol 43, No. 5, pp749-756, 1992.
18. Hall M.S., Topp D.A. and Dover W.D.: Parametric equations for stress intensity factors in weldments. Project Report TSC/MSH/0244, Technical Software Consultants Ltd., Milton Keynes, U.K. 1990
19. C.C. Mohanan, Early Fatigue Crack Growth at Welds, Computational Mechanics Publications, Southampton UK 1995.
20. Fracture Mechanics Proof of strength for engineering components. VDMA-Verlag Frankfurt-M, Germany 2009, ISBN 3-8163-0496-6
21. Fracture mechanics proof of strength for engineering components (Bruchmechanischer Festigkeitsnachweis für Maschinenbauteile), VDMA Frankfurt Germany, 2006, ISBN 3-8163-0514-8
22. BS 7910:2005: Guidance on methods for assessing the acceptability of flaws in metallic structures British Standard Institution, London.Murakami Y.: Stress Intensity Factors Handbook. Pergamon Press, Oxford U.K. 1987
23. Rooke D.P. and Cartwright, D.J.: "Compendium of Stress Intensity Factors." Her Majesty's Stationary Office, London, 1976.
24. Newman J.C. and Raju I.S.: Stress intensity factor equations for cracks in three-dimensional finite bodies. ASTM STP 791 1983, pp. I-238 - I-265
25. Newman J.C. and Raju I.S.: Stress intensity factors for internal surface cracks in cylindrical pressure vessels. Journal of Pressure Vessel Technology, 102 (1980), pp. 342-346.
26. Newman J.C. and Raju I.S.: An empirical stress intensity factor equation for the surface crack. Engineering Fracture Mechanics, Vol 15. 1981, No 1-2, pp. 185-192
27. Frank K.H. and Fisher J.W.: Fatigue strength of fillet welded cruciform joints. J. of the Structural Div., Proc. of the ASCE, Vol 105 (1979) pp. 1727-1740
28. Albrecht P. and Yamada K.: Rapid calculation of stress intensity factors. J. Struct. Div. ASCE, 1977, 103(ST2), 377-389.
29. Maddox S.J. and Andrews R.M.: Stress intensity factors for weld toe cracks, in 'Localized Damage Computer Aided Assessment and Control'
30. Aliabadi M.H., Brebbia C.A. and Cartwright D.J. (Editors). Computational Mechanics Publications, Southamton, ISBN 1 853 12 070 7, co-published with Springer-Verlag, Heidelberg, ISBN 3 540 527 17 6, 1990
31. Hobbacher A.: Stress intensity factors of welded joints. Engineering Fracture Mechanics, Vol 46 (1993), no 2, pp. 173-182, and Vol 49 (1994), no 2, p. 323
32. Maddox S.J.: Fatigue crack propagation in weld metal and HAZ. Metal Constr. 1970, 2(7), 285-289.
33. Jaccard R.: Fatigue crack propagation in aluminium. IIW Doc. XIII-1377-90
34. Nykänen T., Marquis G. and Björk T.: Simplified assessment of weld quality for fatigue loaded cruciform joints. IIW Document XIII-2177-07
35. Pang H.L.J.: A review of stress intensity factors for a semi-elliptical surface crack in a plate and fillet welded joint. IIW Document XIII-1433-91
36. Shen G, Plumtree A, Glinka G.: Weight function for the surface point of semi-elliptical surface crack in a finite thickness plate. Engineering Fracture Mechanics, vol 40, no. 1, pp 167-176, 1991.

37. Albrecht P. and Yamada K.: Rapid calculation of stress intensity factors. J. of Strutural Div. of the ASCE, 1977,103(ST2), 377-389
38. Maddox S.J. and Andrews R.M.: Stress intensity factors for weld toe cracks, in 'Localized Damage Computer Aided Assessment and Control'
39. Aliabadi M.H., Brebbia C.A. and Cartwright D.J. (Editors). Computational Mechanics Publications, Southamton, ISBN 1 853 12 070 7, co-published with Springer-Verlag, Heidelberg, ISBN 3 540 527 17 6, 1990
40. Hobbacher A. Stress Intensity Factors of Welded Joints. Engineering Fracture Mechanics, Vol.46(1993) No 2, pp 173-182, et Vol 49(1994) No 2, p 323
41. Pang H.L.J.: A review of stress intensity factors for a semi-elliptical surface crack in a plate and fillet welded joint. IIW Document XIII-1433-91
42. Shen G, Plumtree A, Glinka G.: Weight function for the surface point of semi-elliptical surface crack in a finite thickness plate. Engineering Fracture Mechanics, vol 40, no. 1, pp 167-176, 1991.

MIX
Papier aus verantwortungsvollen Quellen
Paper from responsible sources
FSC® C105338

If you have any concerns about our products,
you can contact us on
ProductSafety@springernature.com

In case Publisher is established outside the EU,
the EU authorized representative is:
Springer Nature Customer Service Center GmbH
Europaplatz 3, 69115 Heidelberg, Germany

Printed by Libri Plureos GmbH
in Hamburg, Germany